DATE DUE

DEMCO 38-296

Biomedicine and Alternative Healing Systems in America

BIOMEDICINE AND ALTERNATIVE HEALING SYSTEMS IN AMERICA

Issues of Class, Race, Ethnicity, and Gender

Hans A. Baer

THE UNIVERSITY OF WISCONSIN PRESS

The University of Wisconsin Press
2537 Daniels Street
Madison, Wisconsin 53718

www.wisc.edu/wisconsinpress/

3 Henrietta Street
London WC2E 8LU, England

5   4   3   2   1

Printed in the United States of America

Library of Congress Cataloging-in-Publication Data

Baer, Hans A., 1944–
    Biomedicine and alternative healing systems in America :
    issues of class, race, ethnicity, and gender /
    Hans A. Baer.
        pp.   cm.
    Includes bibliographical references and index.
    ISBN 0-299-16690-2 (cloth)
    ISBN 0-299-16694-5 (paper)
        1. Social medicine—United States.   2. Medical anthropology—United
    States.   3. Alternative medicine—United States.   I. Title.
    RA418.3.U6 B34   2001
    306.4′61′0973—dc21   00-012733

Contents

Preface

My scholarly interest in medical pluralism emerged out of the research I conducted from 1977 to 1984 on African American Spiritual churches, first in Nashville, Tennessee, and later in other cities in the South, Midwest, and Northeast (Baer 1984a). As part of this effort, I interviewed eight Spiritual prophets, or advisors, about their religious healing techniques (Baer 1981a). A different medical system caught my attention during the academic year 1979–80 when I held a National Institute of Mental Health (NIMH) postdoctoral fellowship in the Medical Anthropology Program at Michigan State University. While continuing to explore the interface of African American religion and ethnomedicine (Baer 1982), I became intrigued by the history, sociopolitical status, and culture of osteopathic medicine in the United States. Because of my general interest in marginalized groups in American society, particularly Hutterites, Mormons, African American religious groups, communitarian societies, and followers of alternative medical systems, I was particularly struck by the fact that at Michigan State there were two medical schools: the College of Human Medicine, which trains M.D.s, and the College of Osteopathic Medicine, which trains D.O.s, or Doctors of Osteopathy.

I had first encountered osteopathic medicine many years earlier, while I was an engineering student at Pennsylvania State University in the mid-1960s. One of my friends was contemplating switching from engineering to medicine. He spoke to me about possibly applying to the Philadelphia College of Osteopathic Medicine, not because he had a strong interest in osteopathy as an alternative medical system, but because of his rather mediocre GPA. Somehow he had discovered that he had a better chance of being admitted to an osteopathic medical school than to an M.D.-granting school. A few years later I became curious about both osteopathy and chiropractic as a result of reading Martin Gardner's somewhat jaundiced treatment of them in *Fads and Fallacies in the Name of Science* (1957:199–203). In the course of my travels around the country in the early 1970s, I poked around the campuses of the osteopathic colleges in Kansas City, Missouri, and Des Moines, Iowa. At the latter, I struck up a conversation with a few students in the dining area. They confessed that they had not been admitted to M.D.-granting schools and had opted to attend an osteopathic school as a different route into medicine. Simply put, they were interested in becoming "doctors," not "osteopaths" or "osteopathic physicians."

While at Michigan State, I quickly befriended Jim Riley, a medical anthropologist who held a joint appointment in the Medical Anthropology Program and the College of Osteopathic Medicine. He and I had many pleasant conversations about osteopathy, and he opened doors for me into the culture of the profession by introducing me to a number of osteopathic physicians. Jim eventually "went native" by becoming an osteopathic physician himself. Unlike many students, he was interested in osteopathy because he believed that it had the potential to rejuvenate itself as an alternative medical system. Intrigued by this idea, I conducted research that eventually culminated in an article on the organizational rejuvenation of osteopathic medicine in the United States (Baer 1981b). I also met three D.O.s, Myron Beal, John Upledger, and Fred Mitchell, Jr., who acquainted me with British osteopathy. With a generous grant from the National Osteopathic Foundation, I was able to conduct ethnographic and archival research on British osteopathy during the summer of 1983 (Baer 1984b). Unlike American osteopathy, which, as I argue in this book, has evolved into a parallel health care system to conventional medicine, with an emphasis on family practice, British osteopathy remains an alternative medical system.

My study of chiropractic developed in large part as a spin-off from my study of osteopathy. During the course of my research on British osteopathy, it became increasingly apparent to me that its sociopolitical status and scope of practice were quite similar to that of British chiropractic. As a consequence, I decided to visit the Anglo-European College of Chiropractic in Bournemouth and to interview several practicing chiropractors in both England and Edinburgh, Scotland (Baer 1984c). In a similar way, I developed an interest in naturopathy as a spin-off from my work on both osteopathy and chiropractic. Later, during my stint as a visiting professor at the University of California, Berkeley, in spring 1994, I had the opportunity to learn about acupuncture and the holistic health movement.

I first began to contemplate writing this book after publishing an article titled "The American Dominative Medical System as a Reflection of Social Relations in the Larger Society," which appeared in a special issue of *Social Science and Medicine*, "Marxist Approaches in Medical Social Science," guest edited by Howard Waitzkin (Baer 1989). I felt that the article contained the organizing framework for a comprehensive overview of the relationship between biomedicine and a wide array of alternative medical systems in the United States. I began to work more systematically on the subject while I was teaching a course at Berkeley on medical pluralism in North America and Europe. This book represents the culmination of twenty years of research on medical pluralism in American society.

Acknowledgments

Numerous institutions, organizations, and individuals contributed to my understanding of medical pluralism in the United States. I first became immersed in the relationship between biomedicine and osteopathic medicine while an NIMH postdoctoral fellow in the Medical Anthropology Program at Michigan State University. Invitations to lecture at the Texas College of Osteopathic Medicine in Fort Worth, the Canadian Memorial Chiropractic College in Toronto, the Palmer School of Chiropractic, and the Los Angeles College of Chiropractic allowed me to become acquainted with osteopathic physicians and chiropractors in various settings. Visits to John Bastyr University in Seattle, the National College of Naturopathic Medicine in Portland, Oregon, and the Southwestern College of Naturopathic Medicine in Tempe, Arizona, advanced my understanding of American naturopathy. Students in my class on medical pluralism in North America and Europe at the University of California, Berkeley, in spring 1994 provided me with important insights into the holistic health movement and acupuncture in the San Francisco Bay Area through both their mini-ethnographies and their conversations with me on alternative medical systems. The following people in particular have contributed to my insights on alternative medical systems in the United States: Myron Beal, Philip Greenman, Fred Mitchell, Peter Kong-Ming New, Jim Riley, and John Upledger on osteopathic medicine; Alan Adams, Robert Anderson, Ian Coulter, Joe Keating, Caroline Peterson, and Walter Wardwell on chiropractic; Joe Pizzorno, Stephen Sporn, and Retta Ward Stapp on naturopathy; Dana Ullman on homeopathy; Kathy Sanders on massage therapy; Jill Crewes on lay midwifery; Robbie Moreland-Adams and Merrill Singer on Christian Science; Sandra Simmons on Unity; numerous members of Spiritual churches on African American religious healing; Vivian Garrison and Merrill Singer on Puerto Rican *espiritismo*; and George Brandon on *santeria*. I am highly indebted to David Hess at Rensselaer Polytechnic Institute and Merrill Singer at the Hispanic Health Council in Hartford for having read two earlier versions of this book in its entirety. I would also like to thank Louise E.

Robbins for her conscientious efforts as a copy editor. Last, but not least, Rosalie Robertson, senior editor at the University of Wisconsin Press, played an extremely supportive role in facilitating the publication of this book as she did for the publication of my *Recreating Utopia in the Desert: A Sectarian Challenge to Modern Mormonism* (1988) while she was an editor at the State University of New York Press.

Biomedicine and Alternative Healing Systems in America

Introduction

This book provides a historical and sociopolitical overview of medical pluralism in the United States. In capitalist societies, people in different class, racial/ethnic, and gender categories tend to have different ideologies, which are reflected in cultural differences (Navarro 1986:171). I show how these groups have constructed distinctive medical systems to coincide with their diverse views of reality.

The occurrence of medical pluralism itself has been recognized by a fair number of medical anthropologists, who have observed that in complex societies, including the United States, multiple, often antagonistic medical systems tend to coexist. For example, anthropologist Charles Leslie, who has done extensive research on medical pluralism in South Asia, notes that:

> Even in the United States, the medical system is composed of physicians, dentists, druggists, clinical psychologists, chiropractors, social workers, health food experts, masseurs, yoga teachers, spirit teachers, Chinese herbalists, and so on. The health concepts of a Puerto Rican worker in New York City, the curers he consults, and the therapies he receives, differ from those of a Chinese laundryman or a Jewish clerk. Their concepts and the practitioners they consult differ in turn from those of middle-class believers in Christian Science or in logical positivism. (1976:9-10)

Although such social scientists readily recognize the ethnic and even gender dimensions of medical pluralism, however, they tend to ignore or downplay the way in which it exemplifies class relations in the larger society. Conversely, critical social scientists, aside from a few exceptions (Berliner and Salmon 1980; Elling 1981; Frankenberg 1981; Salmon 1984; Singer and Borrero 1984), confine their analyses to the orthodox, or regular, medical system and ignore or at best give fleeting attention to alternative medical systems. I attempt to provide a corrective to this oversight by arguing that the phenomenon of medical pluralism has historically reflected and continues today to reflect class, racial/ethnic, and gender relations in American society.

3

Although the majority of medical practitioners in the nineteenth century were regular physicians, they did not exert clear dominance over alternative practitioners. According to Berliner, two "medical modes of production" co-existed in early nineteenth-century American society: a "domestic mode," in which "medical care was produced and performed as a use value, generally within the family," and a "petty commodity mode," in which medical care assumed exchange value (1982:165). The domestic mode comprised a variety of folk medical systems, including European American folk medicine, African American folk medicine, Native American healing traditions, bone-setting, and home remedies. On the American frontier, these folk systems often borrowed liberally from one another and to some degree coalesced into a syncretic amalgam.

The petty mode of production consisted primarily of regular medicine and homeopathic medicine; both were performed by trained physicians who charged a fee for their services. While regular medicine, characterized by "heroic" procedures such as bleeding, leeching, and strong drugs, had functioned as virtually the sole form of professionalized medicine during the eighteenth century, homeopathy, an "extremely minimalist medicine" (Berliner 1985:39) based on the use of very dilute drugs, found a niche in the competitive marketplace of the new American republic after it was imported from Europe in the mid-1820s. Homeopathy initially appealed to some lower-class people, but its professional orientation transformed it into a fashionable form of medicine for the affluent. The serious economic threat posed by homeopathy's status as a professionalized heterodox medical system was one of the major factors that prompted regular physicians to establish the American Medical Association in 1847. Regular medicine faced challenges from several other heterodox medical systems as well, some of which (e.g., botanic medicine) underwent a professionalization process of their own as the nineteenth century unfolded.

As American capitalism evolved from a competitive to a monopoly form after the Civil War, the corporate class found it necessary to exert control over an increasingly restless populace. Along with the state and education, medicine became yet another hegemonic vehicle by which members of the corporate class indirectly came to legitimate capital accumulation and to filter their view of reality down to the masses. The corporate class acquired an effective tool around the turn of the century, with the development of the germ theory and the transition to "scientific medicine," or "biomedicine," a medical system based on systematic scientific research and controlled experimentation. With its emphasis upon pathogens as the cause of disease, biomedicine provided corporate leaders with a paradigm that allowed them to neglect the social origins of disease while at the same time, in at least some instances, restoring workers back to a level of functional health essential to capital accumulation.

4

The relationship between biomedicine and alternative medical systems has been characterized by processes of annihilation, restriction, absorption, and even collaboration. However, since strategic elites situated in the corporate sector, government, and health foundations ultimately shape health policy, the power of biomedicine is delegated rather than absolute. As Navarro observes, "the medical profession is a stratum of trustworthy representatives to whom the bourgeoisie delegates some of its authority to run the house of medicine" (1986:27). Traditionally, physicians have been given authority to make medical decisions in their various workplaces. Yet, because the state increasingly has come to act as an arena of class struggle and to assume the role of pacifying social dissent and resolving the contradictions of a capitalist society, including those in the health sector, it periodically must make concessions to alternative health practitioners and their clients, who often belong to lower-middle, working, and even lower social classes. Alternative medicine is one form of dissent in the area of health care; another is the formation of self-help groups, whose growth, according to Williams and Calnan "can . . . be seen in terms of a lay resistance to the dominance of medical instrumental rationality over experiential forms of knowledge" (1996:1616). In response to such resistance, corporate and governmental elites involved in health policy decision-making may partially or completely legitimate a particular alternative medical system by licensing its practitioners, certifying its educational institutions, and providing subsidies for patient care and medical care. Through this process of legitimation, some alternative practitioners (e.g., osteopaths, chiropractors, Christian Science practitioners, and folk healers) have been able to override opposition by orthodox medical professionals to their licensing or even provision of services in biomedical settings. Furthermore, the corporate class and its state sponsors may provide support of one sort or other to alternative medical systems if they feel that these systems serve certain functions for them or are cheaper than biomedical therapies.

Patterns of legitimation and even professionalization of various alternatives may illustrate that indeed the dominance of organized biomedicine is limited. They also, however, reflect the growing accommodation by alternative practitioners to a reductionist theory that disease is the result of a few simple causes; a theory that is compatible with both capitalist ideology and the biomedical model of organization. Unless they are part of a major societal transformation, alternative medical systems must accommodate themselves to what Wallace (1956) terms "special interest groups" (e.g., organized regular medicine, corporate and governmental elites, and health policy decision-makers) if they are to survive and prosper. These systems will remain weak even as they grow, according to Saks: "while access to the alternatives to medicine may be expanded, the traditional monopolistic power base of the orthodox profession still seems highly likely to dilute the scope of what is available, even at a time when the profession is coming under ever-greater challenge from the consumer in an increasingly market-based society" (1994:100).

Although much has been written about the wide array of medical systems, both professionalized and popular, that exists in the United States, what has been lacking is a comprehensive overview of this medical pluralism. In providing such an overview, I use as a starting point three significant features of this phenomenon: medical pluralism involves hierarchical relations among medical subsystems; these hierarchical relations tend to mirror the political, economic, and social relationships and divisions of the larger society; and in the American hierarchical medical system, only one subsystem, biomedicine, has come to enjoy preeminence and, with the support of social elites, attempts to exert dominance over subordinate subsystems.

In chapter 1, I examine the pluralistic nature of American medicine in the nineteenth century, looking at various medical systems that arose from several sectors of the populace and acted as challenges to regular medicine. Chapter 2 describes the development of biomedicine into a hegemonic institution, the demise of homeopathy and eclecticism, and the sociopolitical status of biomedicine as the dominative actor in the American medical system. Chapter 3 discusses the emergence of osteopathic medicine as a parallel medical system focusing on primary care. Chapters 4 and 5 focus on the development, philosophical premises, and social organization of three professionalized heterodox medical systems: chiropractic, naturopathy, and acupuncture. In chapter 6, I discuss various aspects of partially professionalized and lay heterodox medical systems within the context of the holistic health movement as well as oppositional and accommodative dimensions of the holistic health movement itself. Chapter 7 examines several Anglo-American religious healing systems, particularly Spiritualism, New Thought groups, Pentecostalism, the charismatic movement, and Scientology. Chapter 8 provides an overview of European American, African American, Haitian American, Hispanic, East Asian, and Native American folk medical systems and shows how they juxtapose elements of protest and accommodation to the larger society. In the conclusion, I consider the attention biomedical physicians are now paying to the holistic health movement, the growing corporate and government interest in alternative medical systems, the persistence of folk medical systems among working-class Americans, particularly those of color, and the potential for developing an authentically holistic and pluralistic medical system in the United States.

1

Nineteenth-Century American Medicine as a Pluralistic System

American medicine during the nineteenth century was highly pluralistic. Regular medicine shared the stage with a wide array of competing and sometimes complementary alternative medical systems, including homeopathy, botanic medicine, eclecticism, hydropathy, Christian Science, osteopathy, and chiropractic. Although regular medicine constituted the most widespread subsystem, it did not completely dominate its rivals economically, politically, or socially.

Much of regular medicinal practice from the colonial era to around 1850 took the form of what medical historians have designated "heroic medicine": physicians relied heavily upon techniques such as bleeding, leeching, blistering, cupping, purging, sweating, and administering toxic and sometimes addictive drugs (Kaufman 1976:57). In the early nineteenth century, various sectors of the American populace began to question these drastic methods of bodily intervention. A number of competitors stepped in to challenge regular medicine's economic, political, and social influence in American society, thus transforming nineteenth-century American medicine into a pluralistic system in which no one medical subsystem was dominant. According to Brown, the regular medical profession lacked power, wealth, and status up until the late nineteenth century:

> Medicine at that time was pluralistic in its theories of disease, technically ineffective in preventing or curing sickness, and divided into several warring sects. Existing professional organizations had virtually no control over the entry of new doctors into the field. Physicians as a group were merely scattered members of the lower professional stratum, earning from several hundred to several thousand dollars a year and having no special status within the population. (1979:5)

This rivalry among "warring sects" within medicine resembled the rivalry manifested by the many religious sects of the time. Indeed, proponents of both regular and alternative, or heterodox, medical systems used religious terminology then as well as later to characterize each other. Medical sectarians viewed regular medicine as a fossilized "orthodoxy" that treated patients with a mechanistic approach. Regular physicians, in turn, branded heterodox groups as "cults," using the same language that orthodox religions used against unorthodox sects (see Reed 1932 for use of this terminology).

Most of the challengers to regular medicine that emerged in nineteenth-century America manifested a metaphysical or religious component, even when their theories of disease centered on natural, rather than supernatural, causes. Homeopathy, Thomsonianism, Grahamism, and hydropathy, which emphasized, respectively, highly dilute drugs, herbal cures, vegetarianism and moderate living, and water treatment, all "resonated with the progressivist and perfectionist tendencies of early nineteenth-century American Protestantism" (Fuller 1989:9). Heterodox systems were often based on vitalism, the view that the body cannot be understood simply in terms of chemical and physical processes, and heterodox practitioners often contrasted their emphasis on vitalism to regular medicine's mechanistic approach. Many heterodox systems drew upon mesmerism, or magnetic healing, a method developed by Franz Anton Mesmer (1734–1815), a Viennese physician (Fuller 1989:38–49). Mesmerists believed that they could realign imbalances in the magnetic fluid, a vital force that coursed through the body, by using magnets or passing their hands over the patient's afflicted areas. Direct linkages between religion and heterodox medicine existed in the case of the new religious sects that arose in the nineteenth century. The Mormons favored botanic medicine, the Seventh-day Adventists hydropathy, and the Swedenborgians and the Christian Scientists homeopathy (Starr 1982:95). Regular medicine was not entirely immune to such influences, however; vitalism, for example, had been a central component of orthodox medicine in the early nineteenth century, and later in the century it "continued to find outlet in the writings of the medical establishment" (Cooter 1988:71).

NINETEENTH-CENTURY REGULAR MEDICINE

The emergence of medical pluralism in nineteenth-century America must be viewed in relation to both the nature of heroic medicine, which was the dominant approach of regular practitioners at the time, and the status of regular medicine as a distinct profession. Regular medicine came to be termed "heroic" because physicians took extraordinary measures to intervene in the healing process and manage the patient's care. William Cullen (1710–1790), of Edinburgh, and his student Benjamin Rush (1746–1813), of Philadelphia, played pivotal roles in the development of this therapeutic method. Cullen criticized his peers "for their timidity in therapeutics and for too much trust in the curative powers of nature" (Berman 1978:77). He advocated treating disease by administering remedies such as calomel, antimony, emetics, purgatives, and opiates, and by bleeding, cupping, blistering, leeching, and prescribing a starvation diet. Physicians often attempted to induce either vomiting or diarrhea as a means of extracting poisonous bodily substances. Some historians have argued that George Washington's death on December 14, 1799, was in large part at the hands of three attending physicians (one of whom had been personally trained by Benjamin Rush) who were considered state-of-the-art practitioners of heroic medicine (Duffy 1976:102). In the second quarter of the nineteenth century many people began to oppose this system of medicine and to seek out homeopaths and botanical practitioners, and by the mid-1850s regular practitioners had also begun to criticize heroic therapy (Rothstein 1987:41). By 1870, regular medical schools had ceased teaching bloodletting and other extreme measures (Kaufman 1971:110–12). Despite the demise of the heroic approach after the Civil War, the practice of regular medicine continued to be primarily allopathic, that is, seeking to counteract or even combat the forces of nature.

Medicine was a relatively open endeavor in colonial America. Individuals could become healers by three different avenues: training in a European medical school or hospital, apprenticeship, or informal education of some sort (Rothstein 1987:25). In colonial and early nineteenth-century America, most regular physicians obtained their medical education through an apprenticeship, a three-year program of study under a practicing physician. Opportunities for formal study in classes and medical schools first became available in the mid-eighteenth century. In the 1750s and 1760s, private instructors began to offer anatomy courses in several northeastern cities (Rothstein 1987: 48). Soon afterwards, organized medical schools were established at the University of Pennsylvania in 1765, at King's College (now Columbia University) in 1767, at Harvard University in 1783, and at Dartmouth College in 1797 (Rothstein 1987:29). The number of regular medical schools increased to six by 1810, 13 by 1820, 22 by 1830, 42 by 1850, 47 by 1860, and 160 by 1900 (Rothstein 1987:49, 92). Many of the medical schools founded in the early nineteenth century, especially those west of the Appalachians, were proprietary, or profit-making, institutions. Funded by student fees and subsidies from states and local communities (Rothstein 1987:31, 36), these schools, which required only a high school diploma, offered opportunities for students in rural areas. According to Kunitz, "many poor boys were able to set up as physicians relatively easily and thereby improve their social status"(1974:20). Before the Civil War, rural medical schools educated approximately one-third of all regular medical students (Rothstein 1987:31).

As heterodox medicine grew in popularity during the early nineteenth century, regular physicians began to form societies and publish journals. Members of local medical societies attempted to reduce competition by cre-

9

ating a fee system and codes of etiquette. Many state medical societies also were established, and in 1847 the American Medical Association (AMA) was founded. Regular medical journals served as forums for denouncing hetero-dox medicine and consolidating orthodox identity. According to Warner, com-petition from medical sects provided a strong impulse for regular physicians to organize:

> Medical orthodoxy in the United States was created with the rise of sectarian-ism. Prior to the emergence of medical sects, a broad spectrum of practition-ers—diverse in social background and intellectual attainment—shared the self-perception of being legitimate, regularly educated practitioners. They seldom questioned each other's regularity . . . .
>
> As sectarian attacks upon regular medicine mounted after the 1820s, however, these physicians continued to reflect upon their relationship to those who were assailing them. The rise of medical sectarianism heightened regular practitioners' awareness of their group identity and its rooting in allegiance to a shared tra-dition. With the strengthening concept of orthodoxy, regular physicians looked for ways of setting themselves apart from heterodox healers and purifying their ranks. (1987:240–41)

In order to restrict competition, the AMA attempted to standardize the re-quirements for medical degrees. The regular medical schools, however, often refused to comply with these efforts; they admitted most applicants who could pay the required fees and did not want to cut into the generation of reve-nue. The AMA also enacted a code of ethics which forbade consultation with heterodox physicians. Although the AMA was able to make it more difficult for heterodox practitioners to obtain positions in the federal government, it was not successful in establishing a monopoly for regular medicine. Homeopaths and eclectics continued to prosper (Starr 1982:91).

Despite strategies such as the formation of the AMA, however, regular medicine remained highly fragmented during much of the nineteenth cen-tury. Up until the end of the century, intra-professional rivalries were com-mon. The medical elite, for example, often looked down on ordinary physi-cians (Starr 1982:89). Some regular physicians belonged to the American Association of Physio-Medical Physicians and Surgeons (est. 1883) and others to the American Association of Physicians and Surgeons (est. 1894) (Burrow 1963:5). In 1886, the AMA "became so embroiled in political squabbles that the more scientifically minded members split off to form a separate learned society"(Starr 1982:91). A little over a decade later, in 1899, yet another rift ap-peared. Twenty M.D.s who opposed the exclusive policies of the AMA formed the American Medical Union in order "to secure the repeal of all medical statutes based on the principles of despotic paternalism" (quoted in Burrow 1963:5). Despite their efforts to monopolize health care, regular physicians were at best able to function as "first among equals" in the pluralistic medical marketplace of nineteenth-century America.

EARLY CHALLENGERS TO REGULAR MEDICINE: HOMEOPATHY, BOTANIC MEDICINE, THE POPULAR HEALTH MOVEMENT, SEVENTH-DAY ADVENTISM, AND SPIRITUALISM

The popularity of heterodox medicine in early nineteenth-century America stemmed in large part from a pervasive dissatisfaction with regular medicine and from the anti-elitist sentiments of the Jacksonian era. In 1873, by the time heroic therapies had been expunged from regular medicine, of the some 50,000 practicing physicians in the United States, 39,219 were regulars, 2,955 homeopaths, 137 hydropaths, 2,857 eclectics, and 4,832 other sorts of practitioners (Haller 1994:164–65). Of these alternatives to regular medicine, homeopathy was, for a time, the most significant.

HOMEOPATHY

Homeopathy was developed by Samuel Hahnemann (1755–1843), a German who studied medicine at both the University of Leipzig and the University of Erlangen. Frustrated by the ineffectiveness of regular medicine, he gave up his practice and began translating both classical and contemporary medical works into German. His reading led him to consider how drugs affect the human body and to develop the first principle of homeopathy, the "law of similars," which posits that like cures like. On the basis of his own experiments, Hahnemann concluded that an efficacious medicine is one that induces in a healthy person symptoms similar to those of the disease for which it is administered. Disease, he believed, was caused by perturbations in the spiritual force that animates and governs the body. Homeopathic doses were designed to strengthen the vital spirit. After becoming an itinerant physician in Germany and Austria, Hahnemann developed a second principle of homeopathy, the "law of infinitesimals," which asserted that the potency of a medicinal substance increases the more it is diluted. Hahnemann's therapy involved considerable personal attention; the homeopathic physician spent a great deal of time taking the patient's history in order to determine the exact set of symptoms. Hahnemann contrasted his system with "allopathy," a term he coined for regular medicine because of its interventionist practices. Homeopathy became extremely fashionable among the nobility and upper class in Europe, and Hahnemann, who died at age 89, enjoyed a long career as a successful and wealthy physician (Kaufman 1971:23–27; Starr 1982:97).

11

Homeopathy diffused to America in the mid-1820s. Hans B. Gram, a Danish American who studied medicine in Denmark, and his disciple, John F. Gray, were the first homeopaths to practice in the United States (Kaufman 1971:28; Kaufman 1988:100). Homeopathy arrived in the United States at a favorable time, according to Haller—"a time when medical men were beginning to question several longstanding procedures, such as bleeding, cupping, heroic dosage, and salivation"(1981:106). Indeed, many homeopathic physicians in the eastern United States were converts from allopathy. The other major source of homeopaths was the immigration of German homeopathic physicians who came to treat German Americans in Pennsylvania and the Midwest (Coulter 1973:101). New York City became the major center of homeopathy in the United States. It was popular throughout the Northeast and the Midwest, but in the South it gained few adherents outside of Virginia and Louisiana (Coulter 1973:110). Homeopathy did not become significant in terms of numbers of physicians until after the 1850s, but by the 1870s and 1880s it constituted the most influential heterodox medical system in the United States (Starr 1982:96–99).

Homeopathy, while initially appealing to some lower-class people, quickly came to be especially popular with affluent people seeking an alternative to regular medicine (Rothstein 1972:160). It also gained a large following among women (Numbers 1978:90). Although a homeopathic "domestic kit," consisting of a guide and infinitesimal medicines, became an essential element in many households, most homeopaths rejected a strong emphasis on the domestic mode of medical production (Numbers 1978:91). This attitude was probably caused by the fact that homeopaths enjoyed high incomes at a time when many regular physicians struggled to earn a livelihood. Regular physicians regarded homeopathy as a threat, according to Duffy, because its early practitioners were converts from orthodox medicine;

> hence the regulars could scarcely ignore the homeopaths as ignorant and unlettered folk practitioners. Further, homeopathy appealed to the middle and upper classes, the main source of income for the regular practitioners. . . . Finally, homeopaths could not be dismissed as empirics [practitioners who adopted a trial-and-error approach] because they offered a rationale for their practice. (1976:116–17)

Like other heterodox medical practitioners, homeopaths quickly divided into various shades of "purists" and "mixers." The purists, or "high" homeopaths, subscribed to the belief that a highly diluted dosage acts as the most potent drug, whereas the mixers, or "lows," administered not only low-potency (less dilute) homeopathic drugs but also allopathic ones. The mixers gained ascendancy by the middle of the nineteenth century. In addition to allopathic procedures and large doses of homeopathic drugs, mixers incorporated other techniques, such as electrotherapy, cold water douches, water baths, and hypnotism, and they no longer believed in Hahnemann's "vital force," which they regarded as unscientific (Kaufman 1971:116–22; Starr 1982:101).

In order to distinguish themselves from alleged homeopathic pretenders, educated homeopaths formed exclusive professional associations. The American Institute of Homeopathy (AIH) was established in 1844, and, the following year, restricted its membership to physicians who had received a regular medical education (Coulter 1973:124–25). In 1880, at about the same time that American homeopathy reached its zenith, the purists left the AIH and established the Internal Hahnemannian Association (Kaufman 1971:121). Since homeopaths had been barred in 1847 from regular medical societies, hospitals, college faculties, and consultations with regular physicians, they established their own institutions. In these endeavors, the homeopathic profession received considerable economic and political support from its wealthy clients and patrons. By 1898 homeopaths had established nine national societies, 33 state societies, 85 local societies, 39 other local organizations, 66 general hospitals, 74 specialty hospitals, and 31 journals (Rothstein 1972: 236). Homeopaths also founded numerous medical schools. The Homeopathic Medical College of Pennsylvania was established in 1848 (Rothstein 1972:232), and by 1900 there were 22 homeopathic colleges in existence (Coulter 1973:450). Homeopaths operated medical schools affiliated with Boston University and with state universities in Michigan, Iowa, Minnesota, Nebraska, California, and Ohio (Rothstein 1972:237).

"Mixers" tended to dominate in homeopathic medical schools and hospitals. Professors in homeopathic colleges were split between "highs" (especially teachers of pharmacology and therapeutics) and "lows" (teachers of anatomy, physiology, and pathology), but, overall, those favoring low-potency doses prevailed, which resulted in a downplaying of Hahnemannian principles (Coulter 1973:443). Coulter (1973:378) argues that economic factors transformed homeopathic hospitals into bastions of low-potency practice. The individual attention that homeopaths favored was extremely difficult to implement in the assembly-line conditions of the hospital and further encouraged the adoption of standardized allopathic remedies. Other boundaries between homeopathy and allopathy continued to disappear. Many regular physicians began to consult with homeopaths, and in the 1880s, homeopaths gained entry into hospitals in Boston and Chicago (Starr 1982:102). In 1899, the AIH redefined a homeopathic physician as "one who *adds* to his knowledge of [regular] medicine a special knowledge of homeopathic therapeutics" (quoted in Brown 1979:89).

BOTANIC MEDICINE AND ECLECTICISM

In addition to homeopathy, other medical systems became popular in early nineteenth-century America. Many can be described in Berliner's terms as "a petty mode of medical production in which individuals begin to sell a skill (medical diagnosis or cure) as a means of livelihood" (1982:163). Botanic medicine in particular appealed to frontier people, farmers, and the growing urban proletariat, or working class. Samuel Thomson (1769–1843), a New Hampshire farmer who founded the popular Thomsonian movement, learned about medicinal herbs from local herb doctors. After successfully treating his family and neighbors, he became a full-time botanic practitioner in 1805. Thomson's system of herbal medicine used over 70 botanicals, including lobelia powder, bayberry root bark, cayenne pepper, ginger, and poplar bark. Based on his theory that disease resulted from the loss of body heat, Thomson devised a procedure that began with steam baths and continued through six prescribed steps, the first of which called for administering lobelia, red pepper, and brandy to heat the body, cleanse the stomach, and induce perspiration. Treatment with emetics, purgatives, enemas, and sweat-producing herbs followed. Thomson patented his healing techniques on March 3, 1813, and authorized his agents to sell "family rights" to his botanic medicine for $20. Through sales of his instruction book, he hoped to fulfill his goal of transforming everyone into his or her own physician. Thomson's *New Guide to Health* sold briskly and was translated into German for use by the Pennsylvania Dutch. Over 100,000 patents had been sold by the 1840s (Haller 1994:37–45, 50).

Thomson's appeal related to the social and political circumstances of nineteenth-century America. The system became an integral part of the Popular Health Movement, which included lay healers, herbalists, artisans, farmers, and working-class people who opposed licensing for regular physicians (Brown 1979:63). The Thomsonians viewed themselves as allies of working people and opponents of the "tyranny of priests, lawyers, and doctors" (Starr 1982:52). Thomsonians also considered themselves in the forefront of the nineteenth-century feminist movement. Botanic medicine was popular among women, who, as practitioners, could perform their traditional role as healers, and, as patients, appreciated being treated by other women (Haller 1994:47–48). Thomson appealed to nationalist sentiment, as well, claiming, for instance, that "domestic herbs were more suited to American constitutions" (Kett 1980:122).

Thomson organized a convention of delegates from Friendly Botanic Societies—local groups of Thomsonians—in Columbus, Ohio, on December 17, 1832. This gathering reportedly constituted the first national meeting of medical professionals ever held in the United States. The third Thomsonian convention in Baltimore in October 1834 passed the "so-called Test Resolution, which stipulated that no member of the convention would use as medicines any animal, mineral, or vegetable poisons; nor would any member bleed, blister, or sell medicines that were kept secret; nor would they sell any article contrary to the principles established by Samuel Thomson" (Haller 1994:59). Despite this pledge to uphold fundamental principles, Thomsonians disagreed on a number of issues, such as whether to found a medical school. Thomson, fearing that the conventions were aggravating internal conflicts, recommended in 1838 that the convention system be dismantled. In response, Alva Curtis (1797–1881), one of Thomson's agents, and his followers formed the Independent Thomsonian Botanic Society. Most state societies aligned themselves with either Thomson or Curtis. In time, Curtis moved beyond Thomson's ideas and drew upon the health reform ideas of Sylvester Graham, mesmerism, and phrenology (Haller 1994:53–59).

Contrary to its initial emphasis on self-care, Thomsonianism became institutionalized and evolved into two interrelated but distinct medical systems: physio-medicalism and eclecticism. "Physios," who drew their inspiration from the ideas of Alva Curtis, eschewed all mineral drugs, relied upon botanical medicines, and emphasized the role of the physician in assisting the "life force" or "vital principle" in every patient (Haller 1997). In 1836 Curtis opened the Botanico-Medical School of Columbus, in Ohio. Curtis later moved the school to Cincinnati, where it became known as the American Medical Institute. Thirteen physio-medical colleges were founded between 1836 and 1911, nine prior to 1861. Other physio-medical schools included the Southern Botanico-Medical College (est. 1839) in Forsyth, Georgia; the Alabama Medical Institute (est. 1844); the Botanico-Medical College of Memphis (est. 1846); the Metropolitan Medical College in New York City (est. 1848); and the Physio-Medical College of Texas (est. 1902) in Dallas (Haller 1997:88–110, 139–46). In time, all of the physio-medical schools closed their doors. The last of these schools, the Chicago Physio-Medical College (est. 1885), was absorbed by the Chicago College of Medicine and Surgery (eclectic) in 1911.

Despite the number of schools founded, physio-medicalism was less successful than other alternative medical systems, according to Haller:

> For all their pretense to reform, the physios did not fare as well as either the homeopaths or the eclectics in the competition for patients and students. . . . Compared with eclectics and homeopaths, they produced fewer physicians and far fewer textbooks and medical journals. Moreover, many physios chose to practice under a banner other than their own, and fewer still sent students to their physio-medical colleges. Because of their smaller numbers, they were forced to rely on eclectic and regular pharmaceutical companies as the principal sources of their medicines. (1997:147–48)

15

In contrast to the physios, the eclectics exhibited a great propensity to incorporate aspects of regular medicine. Indeed, Wooster Beach (1794–1868), founder of eclecticism, was a regular medical school graduate who dubbed himself an "eclectic" because he blended allopathy with other techniques, including those of the Thomsonians, Native American healers, and herbalists (Rothstein 1972:217–18). Beach's three-volume textbook, *The American Practice of Medicine,* was published in 1833. Although his followers relied heavily on botanical drugs, they attempted to replicate the more benign effects of regular medicine. The eclectics, along with the neo-Thomsonians, or physios, expanded their materia medica and relied less and less on steam treatments and emetics and more and more on smallpox vaccination and cathartics (Berman 1956:133). Many eclectics drew upon homeopathy as well.

The principal eclectic society, the National Eclectic Medical Association, was formed in 1848 by a group of eclectic physicians under the original name of the American Eclectic Medical Association (Haller 1994:160). Other eclectic societies came and went. For example, the Reformed Medical Association of the United States held its first and only meeting in 1852 (Berman 1956: 136).

Beach initiated instruction of eclectic principles in 1825 by teaching students in his home. In 1827 he opened the United States Infirmary in New York City, changing its name to the Reformed Medical Academy in 1829, and to the Reformed Medical College of the City of New York the following year (Haller 1994:70). In 1830 he opened another eclectic medical school at Worthington College in Ohio; for 12 years, this school remained the "most prominent institution for the instruction of reformed medical education" (Haller 1994: 76). As a result of financial and organizational problems that closed down Worthington Medical College, several faculty members established, in 1842, the Reformed Medical School of Cincinnati, which was renamed the Eclectic Medical Institute of Cincinnati in 1845 (Haller 1994:82). The Institute essentially served to unite the followers of Beach and the neo-Thomsonians. Joseph R. Buchanan, the dean of faculty at the Institute, incorporated phrenology, neurology, psychometry, or "soul measuring," and Spiritualism into his lectures (Haller 1994:107). After bringing the institute to near financial ruin, he went on to establish the Eclectic College of Medicine in Hamilton County, Ohio, in 1856 and later the College of Therapeutics in Boston in 1881. The Penn Medical University, an eclectic school established in 1853, became the first coeducational medical school in the United States (Rothstein 1972:227; Haller 1994:150). Eclectic colleges in Worcester, Massachusetts, Syracuse and Rochester, New York, and Cincinnati also admitted women (Haller 1994: 153).

Haller asserts that the "eclectic medical schools provided an avenue into the medical profession for men—and women—who lacked the financial and educational opportunities available to those of more material means" (1994: xvii). Some eclectics practiced in the South and West, and there were concentrations in New York, Massachusetts, and Connecticut, but they were most successful in the Midwest (Haller 1994:162). Few became specialists; most midwestern eclectic physicians, according to a study of contributors to the *Eclectic Medical Journal,* practiced in small towns (Rothstein 1972:228). Rothstein suggested that "the eclectics' small-town practices probably enhanced their influence and political power, because [they] were often the only physicians in their communities" (1972:229).

THE HEALTH REFORM MOVEMENT: GRAHAMISM, HYDROPATHY, SEVENTH-DAY ADVENTISM, AND SPIRITUALISM

In addition to Thomsonianism and eclecticism, the health reform movement of the nineteenth century also encompassed Grahamism, hydropathy, Seventh-day Adventism, and Spiritualism. Sylvester Graham (1794–1851), a Presbyterian minister and temperance worker, played a significant role in the health reform movement of the 1830s, especially through lectures he gave in Philadelphia, New York, and Boston on hygiene, sexual moderation, and vegetarianism. Graham believed that Americans were suffering from an increased incidence of disease and nervousness because they ignored the constitutional laws of nature, and he developed a complex theory of physiology that depicted the human body as a fragile organism vulnerable to overstimulation (Nissenbaum 1980:4). He advocated a vegetarian diet that also curtailed dairy products and stimulants (such as coffee and tea) and emphasized the importance of sexual restraint, rest, exercise, cleanliness, loosely fitting clothes, and the avoidance of medicines (Numbers 1992:52–53). As part of his program of dietary reform, Graham developed "Graham bread" and the still popular "Graham cracker." He and his associates, particularly William A. Alcott, maintained that a physician should function as a health educator (Riska 1985:24). They believed that regular physicians failed in their calling because they advanced their own interests rather than those of their patients. The principles of Grahamism found further expression within both hydropathy and Seventh-day Adventism, and many became standard ideas in an enduring health consciousness that is part of counterculturalism in America.

Hydropathy emerged in central Europe as an assortment of water treatments devised by Vincent Priessnitz (1799–1851), a Silesian peasant, who opened a hydropathic spa in 1826. Priessnitz viewed disease as a systemic disorder resulting from a disruption in the human relationship with the natural environment. Hydropaths rejected drugs of every variety, whether botanic or mineral, in large or small doses, as well as bleeding, blistering, cupping, and purging; instead, they placed trust in natural cures such as water treatment, fresh air, sunshine, exercise, and proper (often vegetarian) nutrition (Weiss and Kemble 1967:5; Cayleff 1988:85). As Albanese aptly observes, "for hydropaths, the virtues of pure water occupied the space that herbs and remedies occupied for Thomsonians and homeopaths" (1990:136).

This new medical system was introduced into the United States during the 1840s by regular and homeopathic physicians, some of whom had studied methods of cold water therapy in Europe. Joel Shew, a regular physician who was one of the first American hydropaths, prescribed exercise and a rigid version of the Graham diet (Nissenbaum 1980:149). Russell Trall, also a regular physician, established one of the first water-cure establishments in 1844 and founded the New York Hydropathic School in 1853. He incorporated Grahamism, massage, electrotherapy, exercise, and fresh-air therapy into his system, which he termed "hygeio-therapy." Shew and Trall both served as editors of the *Water-Cure Journal* and wrote widely on health issues (Weiss and Kemble 1967:18–28, 35–36). Another prominent hydropath, Thomas Low Nichols, a graduate of the New York University Medical School, helped to establish the American Vegetarian Society and the American Hygienic and Hydropathic Association of Physicians and Surgeons (Sokolow 1983:127). In 1851 he and his wife, Mary Gove, established the American Hydropathic Institute, a hydropathic medical school, in New York City (Weiss and Kemble 1967:33).

Hydropathy was the first American medical system to underscore the importance of diet, rest, and exercise in the prevention and cure of disease. At the height of its appeal, from 1840 to 1870, there were over 200 hydropathic spas, or cures, many run by physicians, and several water-cure journals. With its emphasis on human perfectibility and social uplift, hydropathy "appealed not only to individualistic and self-seeking strains in American thought but also to gender-specific and culturally valued community bonds, responsibility to others, and continuity in relationships" (Cayleff 1988:83). It catered largely to the urban upper and middle classes but also gave special emphasis to the role of women as providers and consumers of health care, a pattern manifested by the fact that approximately one-fifth of professional hydropaths were women (Numbers 1978). Water cures provided middle-class women with a communal sanctuary from the restrictions of their socially prescribed gender role (Cayleff 1988:92). Hydropathy functioned more on the fringes of regular medicine than as a heterodox medical system per se. Water-cure establishments generally were operated by reform-oriented regular physicians who were assisted by nurses and other support personnel (Weiss and Kemble 1967).

Hydropathy nearly disappeared after Trall's death in 1877, but it underwent a revival in the 1890s in the form of Kneippism, a system of water treatment developed by Father Kneipp, an Austrian priest. Kneippism soon expanded to embrace other natural therapies and was rechristened "naturopathy" by Benedict Lust, leader of the American naturopathic movement (Weiss and Kemble 1967:100–107). In contrast to the situation in the United States, where hydropathy became subsumed under naturopathy, in Germany and other parts of central Europe it continues to be a viable therapeutic modality, with an elaborate network of spas, or *Kurs*.

Hydropathy influenced other therapeutic approaches, especially Seventh-day Adventism. Ellen G. White (1827–1915), the prophetess of Seventh-day Adventism, was a staunch advocate of hydropathy and incorporated many ideas from this and other branches of the health reform movement into her religious sect. Indeed, Fuller even goes so far as to describe Seventh-day Adventism as an "extension of Grahamism" (1989:33). Following a series of visions on healthful living that began in 1848, White began to speak out against tobacco, tea, coffee, rich food, extravagant dress, and uncleanliness. She became an even more ardent advocate of health reform after an encounter with hydropathy in 1863 (Numbers 1992:38–44, 77–85). According to Numbers (1992:86), "for most Adventists, acceptance of health reform meant principally three things: a vegetarian diet, two meals a day, and no drugs or stimulants."

In 1866, White opened the Western Health Reform Institute in Battle Creek, Michigan. John Harvey Kellogg, the first Seventh-day Adventist to become a physician, aimed to transform this water-cure establishment into a respectable medical center by establishing the Medical and Surgical Sanitarium in 1878 (Numbers 1992:126). The church continued to sponsor institutions for medical treatment and education. By 1900, Adventist-run medical centers existed in Portland, Oregon; Boulder, Colorado; Copenhagen; and Sydney, Australia, and in 1910, Adventists established the College of Medical Evangelists in Loma Linda, California. By 1970 the church was operating a global network of 329 medical facilities (Numbers 1992:186, 199–201). Seventh-day Adventist hospitals and colleges, where strict dietary regimes are still followed, have provided researchers with sites for empirical studies that, according to Bergman (1995:43), "constituted an important factor in the modern emphasis on diet as an important means in dealing with many major health concerns."

Like Seventh-day Adventism, American Spiritualism incorporated concepts from the nineteenth-century health reform movement. American Spiritualism can be traced to three sources: the séances conducted by the Fox sisters starting on March 31, 1848, at Hydesville, New York; the teachings of Andrew Jackson Davis; and the widespread popularity of mesmerism. Although the "rappings" received by the Fox sisters propelled Spiritualism into a mass phenomenon, many of the intellectual ideas underpinning the movement were delineated by Andrew Jackson Davis (1826–1910), the "Pough-

19

keepsie Seer," who claimed inspiration from the Greek physician Galen and from Emanuel Swedenborg, a renowned Swedish scientist and mystic. Davis started to heal by prescribing cures after visualizing the inner organs of patients (Moore 1977:10–11). He published *The Principles of Nature* in 1847, a year before the beginning of the Fox séances. During the 1850s, he became the foremost spokesperson for the Spiritualist movement, and he later obtained doctorates in medicine and anthropology from the United States Medical College of New York, an eclectic institution (Delp 1987:109). Spiritualism spread rapidly in the Northeast, the South, and the Midwest, with New Orleans, Chicago, and Cincinnati becoming major centers (Nelson 1969: 13–17). According to Nelson, "Spiritual Circles developed not only in the cities and villages of the settled states of America but also in the camps and settlements in the undeveloped territories of the west, and a number of well-known mediums braved the dangers of these lawless frontier districts to spread knowledge of the movement" (1969:17). Spiritualism achieved its peak in the 1850s, went into decline during the Civil War, and then experienced modest growth in the late nineteenth century (Goldfarb and Goldfarb 1978: 26). It was closely associated with various social movements, particularly the women's rights movement, as well as certain communitarian ventures such as Brook Farm and Hopedale (Braude 1989). Spiritualism attracted a number of prominent supporters, including Horace Greeley, James Fenimore Cooper, William Cullen Byrant, Nathaniel P. Tallmadge, governor of the Wisconsin Territory, and Abraham Lincoln.

Spiritualist congregations began to appear in the late 1850s. Whether or not they exhibited Christian elements, the delivery of messages from the spirit realm constituted the central feature of Spiritualist services. Although they frequented group meetings, Spiritualists tended to eschew the establishment of centralized associations with well-defined doctrinal guidelines. The National Organization of Spiritualists, which claimed to be affiliated with 80 local churches, held a convention in Chicago in 1864 but collapsed several years later. The first permanent Spiritualist organization in the United States, the National Spiritualist Association (est. 1893), was established primarily to counter legal restrictions that had been placed on mediums (Moore 1977:46, 66–67).

Many Spiritualists became healers, borrowing from mesmerism the belief that entranced individuals could heal disease. Although some mediums prescribed medicines, they avoided purgatives, stimulants, and narcotics, and opposed regular medicine:

> Spiritualists incorporated heterodox healing into an integrated worldview that added a critique of the medical establishment to their critiques of the establishment in religion, politics, and society. Spiritualists opposed orthodox medicine

with the same fervor with which they opposed orthodox theology, and with some of the same arguments. Because they viewed each individual as embodying the image of God and the laws of nature, they viewed health, like godliness, as the natural condition of human beings, which only misguided human intervention could destroy. (Braude 1989:144)

Spiritualism offered an avenue for women to become medical practitioners. Most medical mediums were women, and, despite their quarrel with regular medicine, Spiritualists also encouraged women to become physicians. Indeed, a number of Spiritualists were involved in the establishment of the Woman's Medical College in Philadelphia (Braude 1989:148–51). Spiritualists also promoted health reforms such as dress reform, gymnastics, temperance, vegetarianism, and water cure, that "aimed at freeing women from socially constructed restrictions on their physical motion and development" (Braude 1989:151).

LATER CHALLENGERS TO REGULAR MEDICINE: CHRISTIAN SCIENCE, OSTEOPATHY, AND CHIROPRACTIC

Following the Civil War, at the same time that regular physicians were beginning to consolidate their position by lobbying for licensing laws, and homeopaths and eclectics were incorporating more and more aspects of regular medicine into their treatment regimens, several new alternative medical systems appeared in the United States.

CHRISTIAN SCIENCE AND NEW THOUGHT

Christian Science constituted the most organized manifestation of New Thought, a nineteenth-century movement that stressed mind cure, or metaphysical healing. Proponents of New Thought believed that mind could prevail over matter and drew upon concepts from Swedenborgianism, Eastern mysticism, Judeo-Christianity, and Spiritualism (Schoepflin 1988:197). Phineas Parkhurst Quimby (1802–1866), a dabbler in esoteric ideas who cured himself of neurosis through self-hypnotism, served as a pivotal figure in the development of New Thought. He and a partner began to work as healers around Portland, Maine, using mesmerism to determine what remedies to prescribe or to effect cures (Meyer 1965:33–34; Fuller 1989:58–59). Mesmerism, according to Albanese, was a doctrine that taught

> that an invisible fluid provided the vehicle for the "mutual influence between the Heavenly bodies, the Earth and Animate Bodies." The fluid, permeating all living things, provided a medium for them. . . . the presence of the fluid in a balanced

21

ebb-and-flow pattern guaranteed health and vitality, whereas interruptions resulted in what we know as illness. Bathed in this fluid (and, thus material) atmosphere, humans were always in touch with unseen forces that shaped their lives and destinies. Therefore, when illness struck, the magnetic doctor acted as hero-priest, using his or her innate animal magnetism to alter the flow of the invisible fluid—to unblock the obstruction—so that a steady supply of the life-force could reach the ailing person. (1990:108)

Eventually, Quimby came to rely exclusively on mental suggestion rather than mesmerism or drugs as a means for healing illness. In 1869 the Reverend Warren Evans, one of Quimby's patients, published *The Mental Cure*, the first published work of the New Thought movement (Meyer 1965:34).

Mary Baker Eddy (1821–1910), one of Quimby's patients, announced in 1866 that God had revealed to her the "key" by which to heal herself of an injury from a fall that physicians had declared incurable. Since childhood, Eddy had suffered from frequent colds, problems with her lungs and liver, back, and stomach, as well as anxiety and depression. When she failed to find relief from regular physicians, she experimented with self-help remedies and Grahamism and visited homeopaths. She also sought treatment with Quimby, who had a profound impact upon her thinking about health and disease. In 1866 the pains from her fall disappeared after she discovered, while reading in the Bible about Jesus's healings, what she termed the "healing Truth" of Christian Science (Schoepflin 1988:193–94).

Eddy asserted that there is "no Life, Substance, or Intelligence in matter. That all is mind and there is no matter" (quoted in Schoepflin 1988:195). Viewing material reality, including disease and sin, as illusory, she maintained that "mental healing" restores health by eradicating this misconception. Christian Science took homeopathy's administration of infinitesimal dosages to its extreme by eliminating drugs altogether. Christian Science as a religious healing system claimed to eradicate all manner of disease through spiritual power.

Under Eddy's authoritarian leadership and relentless drive, Christian Science grew into an elaborate religious system with a strong emphasis on healing. In addition to drawing upon Quimby's work, Eddy incorporated ideas from transcendentalism, Swedenborgianism, and Spiritualism. She published the influential textbook *Science and Health* in 1875, became the pastor of a group of 26 students in 1879, established the Massachusetts Metaphysical College, which provided instruction in Christian Science healing, in 1881, and started the *Journal of Christian Science* in 1883. A setback occurred in 1888, however, when a Christian Science practitioner was indicted for the death of a mother and child during a birth she had been attending. Although the practitioner was acquitted, the case raised a scandal. Eddy did not support the practitioner and declared that in the future physicians should assist with childbirth cases. Her actions led to internal dissension, and she responded by dissolving the Christian Science Association, the Massachusetts Metaphysical College, the Church of Christ, Scientist, and the National Scientist Association. When she reorganized the sect in 1892, Eddy created a highly centralized Mother Church in Boston, which was administered by a hand-picked bureaucratic apparatus. She reduced the authority of local leaders by limiting their terms of office and controlled practitioners by making their continued practice dependent upon their adherence to the regulations of the organization (Schoepflin 1988:196–99, 203–5). By 1900, the Church of Christ, Scientist, claimed to encompass nearly 500 congregations in North America and Europe (Gottschalk 1988:911).

Christian Science found its greatest appeal among professional and business people, and especially among upper- and middle-class women who rejected the restrictive lifestyle that male physicians and society as a whole prescribed for them. Christian Science made the role of religious healer or practitioner a central aspect of its political-religious hierarchy. As Fox observes, Christian Science "during its formative years—the 1880s and 1890s— assumed the character of an unconscious protest movement for middle-class women who found the practitioner's role an interesting and socially acceptable alternative to the stifling Victorian stereotypes then current" (1989:98). Christian Science also recast the concept of God the Father in Christianity into a father-mother god. During a period when the regular medical profession placed tremendous barriers upon the admission of women into its ranks, the fact that 90 percent of the 3,156 Christian Science practitioners in 1901 were female strongly suggests that Christian Science provided an alternative avenue for obtaining the prestige that healing in all societies commands (Haller 1981:139). Tucker has pointed out that

> as a professional opportunity for women, Christian Science healing was attractive and accessible. With just a few weeks of formal training, curists could list themselves in the *Journal*, stock their homes or rented offices with authorized books for sale, take subscriptions for church periodicals, and see paying clients. Along with the income and entrepreneurial satisfactions, the curists' work brought them influence and prestige within their church communities. (1994:81)

Since Christian Scientists did not administer drugs, perform surgery, or manipulate or touch the patient, it appears that regular physicians regarded them as less threatening economically than were other heterodox practitioners.

Various other New Thought healing groups also developed during the late nineteenth century, including Unity, Divine Science, and Religious Science. Myrtle Fillmore (1845–1931) and her husband Charles Fillmore (1854–1948) cofounded the Unity School of Christianity in 1887 after they had been exposed to Christian Science in Kansas City. The Fillmores organized Unity largely through a number of magazines and, in 1890, established a prayer min-

23

istry which emphasized mental healing. Although Unity does not deny the existence of a physical reality, it teaches that the human mind can exert a great deal of influence on the outcome of events and problems, including disease (Meyer 1965:40–41). Malinda Cramer founded a similar sect in 1888 when she chartered the Home College of Divine Science in San Francisco with the aim of teaching the "Christ Method of Healing" (Judah 1967:195). Divine Science teaches that emotional problems and false thinking induce disease in the body and that healing entails becoming conscious of God's omnipresence within oneself.

Christian Science and other New Thought religious healing systems emerged in the post–Civil War era—a period of increasing industrialization and urbanization. These religions, which appealed primarily to the middle classes rather than to the most impoverished segments of society, provided opportunities to recapture the serenity associated with small-town life. Whereas the industrial capitalist social order made the real world appear chaotic and brutal, New Thought allowed its adherents to find tranquillity by relying upon their inner resources. It also permitted them to either deny the reality of the external world or at least downplay its significance in their lives.

OSTEOPATHY

In contrast to Christian Science, which found its greatest appeal among certain segments of New England petit-bourgeois society, osteopathy and chiropractic, the two other major heterodox medical systems of late nineteenth-century America, reflected the aspirations of midwestern populism. As systems of medicine centered on physical manipulation, they both posited commonsense, mechanical, and reductionist etiologies that were congruent with the pragmatic values of rural American society (McCorkle 1975).

Osteopathy was founded in the 1860s by Andrew Taylor Still (1828–1917), the son of a Methodist minister and a dabbler in mesmerism and Spiritualism, in response to what he perceived to be the excesses of regular medicine (Trowbridge 1991). Although Still was briefly enrolled at the Kansas City College of Physicians and Surgeons in 1860 (Booth 1924), most of his medical training took place as his father's apprentice. He became disenchanted with regular medicine when it failed to prevent the death of three of his children from meningitis. Based upon detailed anatomical investigations, Still concluded that many, if not all, diseases are caused by faulty articulations or "lesions" in various parts of the musculoskeletal system. Such dislocations produce disordered nerve connections which in turn impair the proper circulation of the blood and other body fluids. In his private practice, Still began to rely more and more upon manipulation as a form of therapy. He strongly opposed the use of drugs, vaccines, serums, and modalities such as electrotherapy, radiology, and hydrotherapy. In essence, Still synthesized some of the major components of magnetic healing and bonesetting into a unified medical system. Still's system also had a religious component; he viewed osteopathy as "God's law" and the body as a God-given machine (Gevitz 1982).

After Still was refused permission to present his ideas at Baker University in Baldwin, Kansas (an institution that his father and brothers had helped to establish), he established a base of operations in Kirksville, Missouri, where he applied his concepts in private practice from 1874 to 1892. He reported that on June 22, 1874, he "flung to the breeze the banner of Osteopathy" (Still 1908). Still diligently worked as an itinerant physician who spread the osteopathic message from town to town in Missouri.

Along with William Smith, a graduate of the University of Edinburgh Medical School, Still established the American School of Osteopathy in Kirksville in September 1892. Smith, who served as the first lecturer in anatomy at the school, had impeccable credentials, which provided early osteopathy with a needed aura of legitimacy. The early faculty of the American School of Osteopathy included several other physicians with degrees from both regular and homeopathic colleges.

Osteopathy appealed to thousands of ordinary rural and small-town people, particularly those who were suffering from chronic spinal or joint dysfunctions. According to Cohen,

> Dr. Still took pride in making osteopathy available to everyone including the uneducated under classes. . . . During its early years, osteopathy welcomed even patients who could not pay, as they provided osteopaths with opportunities to demonstrate the movement's altruism and to "Spread the Word." Thus, osteopathy extended to those unable to secure a medical education or treatment elsewhere a medical alternative which was available and eager to have them. (1983: 82)

The opening of an additional 17 osteopathic schools between 1895 and 1900 offered many individuals of humble origins the hope of becoming medical practitioners (Albrecht and Levy 1982:74). Among those enrolled in the early osteopathic schools were also some regular physicians who desired to learn osteopathic manipulation theory (OMT) as an adjunct to their own practices. Most regular physicians, however, were hostile to osteopathy. Despite the opposition of these physicians, who often aligned themselves with homeopathic and eclectic physicians on the matter, osteopaths, with the support of satisfied patients and patrons, quickly acquired at least limited practice rights in most states during the 1890s and the first decade of the twentieth century. Limited practice rights allowed osteopaths to administer OMT and other naturopathic techniques but forbade them from prescribing drugs and performing surgery—procedures that Still and some of his followers eschewed, in any case (Gevitz 1982:41–43).

Despite Still's staunch critique of regular medicine, many of his followers favored blending it with osteopathy. A rather unusual linkage between osteopathy and regular medicine was created at the short-lived Columbian School of Osteopathy. This institution was started by Marcus Ward, a major stockholder and vice-president of the American School of Osteopathy. When personal differences developed between Ward and Still, Ward went off to obtain an M.D. from the University of Cincinnati. In 1897, he returned to Kirksville to establish his own school. Ward not only claimed to be the "co-founder of osteopathy" but also asserted that he had originated "True Osteopathy"—a combination of OMT, surgery, and materia medica. After completion of the Doctor of Osteopathy (D.O.) degree, Columbian students could matriculate for an additional year in order to earn an M.D. (Gevitz 1982:46–47). Although the Columbian School closed in 1901, its existence illustrates the strong tendency toward incorporating allopathic medicine, or "mixing," that has existed since the early years of osteopathy.

CHIROPRACTIC

Like osteopathy, chiropractic blended together elements from various healing and metaphysical systems. Daniel David Palmer, the founder of chiropractic, had experience with Spiritualism, mesmerism, and other esoteric philosophies, and identified God with an "Innate Intelligence" or "Life Force" (Albanese 1986:495). Palmer opened a magnetic healing office in Burlington, Iowa, and later in Davenport, Iowa. He administered his first "spinal adjustment" in Davenport in September 1895, when he cured an African American janitor of a 17-year deafness. Palmer claimed that he had learned of the efficacy of spinal adjustment in treating disease from Dr. Jim Atkinson of Davenport, who was aware of the use of such manipulations in antiquity. Palmer argued that disease emanates from "subluxations," or spinal misalignments. These subluxations result in interference with neural transmission, which in turn triggers dysfunctions in the internal organs. Spinal adjustment restores the normal "nerve force," and health ensues. Palmer began to offer instruction at the Palmer Infirmary and Chiropractic Institute in 1898.

While D. D. Palmer claimed to be the "Discoverer" of chiropractic, his flamboyant son, Bartlett Joshua Palmer (1882–1961), known as "B. J.," clearly was the "Developer" of this new heterodox medical system. Under B. J.'s astute management, the Palmer School grew into "one of the largest institutions that trained health practitioners in the United States, graduating its first 'One Thousand Class' in 1921" (Wardwell 1982:215). B. J. purchased the school from his father in 1907 and turned it into the "Fountainhead," or "Mecca," of the chiropractic profession. Chiropractic probably succeeded so well as an alternative medical system because it reflected the values of middle America:

> It was founded in the Midwest by a Midwesterner, and provides a good fit with several aspects of rural Iowa culture. Rejecting the physicians' complicated and not altogether complete theory of the multiple causation of disease, it offers a "common-sense," single-cause theory that is capable of effective presentation by mechanical analogy. The chiropractic system also upholds the sanctity of the human body and makes use of the healing power of the laying on of hands—two things calculated to appeal to regular Christian teaching. (McCorkle 1975:410)

Given the rivalry that developed between osteopathy and chiropractic, both of which relied on physical manipulation, it is not surprising that many osteopaths asserted that chiropractic was a bastardized version of osteopathy. Chiropractors vehemently objected, and D. D. Palmer himself wryly stated in *The Chiropractor's Adjustor* (1910) that he was "more than pleased to know that our cousins, the osteopaths, are adopting chiropractic methods and advancing along scientific and philosophical lines" (quoted in Gibbons 1980: 13). Arthur Hildreth (1942:45), a member of the first graduating class at the American School, claimed that Palmer received treatments from Still himself, as well as from many of Still's students. Gibbons, a sympathetic but objective historian of chiropractic, maintains:

> It is more than probable that the senior Palmer made the trip [to Kirksville] on several occasions. . . . Charles Still, a son of the founder of osteopathy, contended that Palmer had even been a guest in Still's home. Several Missouri chiropractors who visited the original Still homestead on the campus of what is now the Kirksville College of Osteopathic Medicine had reported seeing D. D.'s name in the guest book in the early 1890s. The younger Still also wrote that an osteopath by the name of Obie Stother had passed on the manipulative techniques of the Old Doctor to the senior Palmer. (1980:13)

Of course, neither Still nor Palmer was the first to view the well-balanced spine as the locus of health. As Lomax observes, both the story and the practice of osteopathy and chiropractic "depended upon concepts acceptable to many eminent nineteenth-century medical practitioners" (1975:15). Osteopathy, in particular, drew upon the notion of "spinal irritation"—the concept that nervous conditions are related to faulty anatomical structures (Schiller 1971:250).

Furthermore, although the connections between the ancient art of bonesetting and both osteopathy and chiropractic remain obscure, techniques for adjusting or manipulating vertebrae and their associated musculature were common on the American frontier. Just as Still relied heavily upon mag-

27

netic healing and bonesetting to develop his form of manipulative therapy, so Palmer merged his earlier interest in magnetic healing with art of bonesetting and with some approaches that he may have picked up from the osteopaths. Osteopaths and chiropractors engaged in a greater cross-fertilization of ideas and techniques than most of them have cared to admit.

THE RELATIONSHIP BETWEEN REGULAR MEDICINE AND ITS COMPETITORS

Licensing regulations or the lack thereof have played a crucial role in the development of American medicine and its constituent medical systems. The history of the licensing of medical practitioners has followed a tumultuous and contradictory course. New York City implemented the first licensure law in the American colonies in 1760 (Duffy 1976:175), and by the end of the eighteenth century, regular physicians had persuaded legislatures in many colonies or states to restrict or prohibit the practices of herbal healers. After the American Revolution, state legislatures extended licensing authority to regular medical societies. Licensing regulations proved to be ineffective, however, because they failed to set up educational standards and to prevent unlicensed practitioners from violating the law (Starr 1982:44–47). Furthermore, as Starr observes, the fragmentary nature of the regular medical profession contributed to the ineffectiveness of licensing laws:

> Neither the top ranks of physicians nor the bottom had a strong interest in effective medical licensing. The less educated practitioners, who had never been to medical school or had never graduated or held degrees of doubtful quality, feared the laws would be used to exclude them. The elite, on the other hand, stood to gain very little from their enactment. (1982:90)

The Popular Health Movement contributed to the repeal of these laws in almost all states during the 1830s and 1840s; its adherents claimed that the laws were elitist and monopolistic and conflicted with the Jacksonian emphasis upon democracy. Health reformers might well have agreed with George Bernard Shaw's assertion that "all professions are conspiracies against the laity" (from *The Doctor's Dilemma* [1906], quoted in Gross 1966:39). By 1849 only New Jersey, Louisiana, and the District of Columbia still had medical licensing laws (Kaufman 1976:68).

Despite the lack of licensing laws between the 1840s and 1870s, regular physicians continued to attack heterodox medical practitioners. Oliver Wendell Holmes, a renowned physician and literary figure, ridiculed homeopathy in 1842 in two influential lectures, later published, titled "Homeopathy, and Its Kindred Delusions" (Kaufman 1971:35–41). Regular physicians dis-

28

missed homeopathic successes by ascribing them to the placebo effect, the power of suggestion, dietary regulations, or natural healing processes. Some asserted that homeopaths administered full-strength drugs rather than the dilute preparations they claimed to use (Coulter 1973:173–74). Despite the inability of the AMA to create a monopoly in the nineteenth century, the association made it "increasingly more difficult for an allopath to adopt homeopathy and remain a member of an orthodox society" (Kaufman 1971:61–62). In addition to barring homeopaths from medical societies, the regular medical profession denied them privileges at regular hospitals, excluded them from many boards of health, and forbade them from teaching in regular medical schools (Rothstein 1972:232–34).

Some regular physicians, however, were willing to cooperate with their homeopathic rivals, many of whom had adopted allopathic treatment regimens; this cooperation apparently served as a strategy of absorbing homeopathy into orthodox medicine. Some members of the Medical Society of the County of New York believed that the AMA's consultation clause, which forbade regular physicians from consulting with heterodox practitioners, "had become an outmoded instrument which prevented physicians from following the dictates of their consciences" (Kaufman 1971:126). The Medical Society of the State of New York appointed a committee that studied the AMA code and recommended a new code which did away with the consultation clause. *The Hahnemannian Monthly*, however, regarded the new code as an effort to co-opt homeopathic physicians into regular medicine (Kaufman 1971:139).

The proliferation of new heterodox medical systems in the late nineteenth century caused concern in the regular medical profession (Burrow 1963:2–6). Beginning in the 1870s, stronger state medical societies emerged and lobbied hard for the establishment of medical examining boards that would set rigorous standards for licensing physicians. By 1893, 18 states required that applicants pass a qualifying examination and another 17 states demanded a diploma from a regular medical school as a requirement for practice. Initially, many states created separate licensing boards for regular physicians, homeopaths, and eclectics. The existence of independent sectarian licensing boards was a source of much vexation to the AMA. Lobbying by the regular medical profession prompted several states to consolidate their multiple boards into single composite boards. Regular physicians conceded to the representation of homeopaths and eclectics on single boards as a means of countering the rise of osteopathy and chiropractic. Needless to say, these boards were dominated by regular practitioners, who were generally in the majority. Of the 45 states with licensing boards around 1900, three states had a single licensing board consisting exclusively of regular physicians; seven states had two or more independent licensing boards, each representing a different medical system; five had a single licensing board, with two or more examining boards for each medical system; and 20 had a single licensing board comprising representatives from various medical systems. Ten states had some other type of licensing board, such as a state board of health, which was authorized to license physicians (Rothstein 1972:307–9).

Although American medicine constituted a relatively pluralistic phenomenon during much of the nineteenth century, some heterodox medical systems, particularly homeopathy and eclecticism, had come increasingly to resemble regular medicine. While the alternative medical systems that appeared during the first half of the nineteenth century, such as homeopathy, eclecticism, Grahamism, hydropathy, and Spiritualism, tended to decline in popularity toward the end of century, those that appeared in the post–Civil War era, such as Christian Science, osteopathy, and chiropractic, survived and prospered as the country entered the twentieth century. These successful heterodox medical systems, however, were not able to prevent the transformation of regular medicine into biomedicine—a system that came to overshadow its competitors in prestige and social influence.

2

The Rise of the American Dominative Medical System under Corporate Capitalism

Regular medicine was transformed into a commodity form in the fullest sense of the term during the late nineteenth century, a process that reflected the rise of industrial capitalism and the wide-ranging impact of this development in Western society. At the same time, medical practitioners attempted to legitimize themselves by appealing to science:

> In the 1890s in the United States, a new mode of medical practice began to emerge. It differentiated itself from allopathy and homeopathy by claiming to be 'scientific' and began to call itself 'scientific medicine,' to benefit from . . . the good-will associated with the word science. (Berliner 1982:168)

Conventional, or regular, medicine in its new guise held itself to be above sectarianism—a view that many medical historians and social scientists accept (Rothstein 1972). The emerging alliance around the turn of the twentieth century between the AMA, which consisted primarily of elite practitioners and medical researchers based in prestigious universities, and the emergent industrial capitalist class ultimately permitted regular medicine to transform itself into biomedicine and to establish political, economic, and ideological dominance over rival medical systems. Some alternative medical systems have managed to persist and are enjoying a resurgence in popularity, but their continued existence depends on their willingness to bend to the biomedical model.

THE RISE OF BIOMEDICINE AS A HEGEMONIC SYSTEM

Changes in the structure and membership of the AMA in the early twentieth century enabled it to undertake or sponsor specific actions that secured the dominance of regular medicine. Despite its self-proclaimed status as the "voice of medicine," the AMA remained a relatively small organization during the nineteenth century. According to Rothstein,

31

In 1900, only 8,400 of the over 100,000 regular physicians in the nation were members. Around the same time, only about 25,000 physicians belonged to all state and local societies affiliated with the AMA. Furthermore, about 40 percent of the AMA's membership in 1900 resided in seven states situated close to the association's Chicago headquarters. The AMA was, in fact, more a regional than a national organization. (1972:317)

Although the AMA was a stronghold of private physicians during its first 50 years, its leadership was taken over by a small institutionally based elite around 1900. Berliner asserts that early in the twentieth century, the AMA came to function as "an organization of scientists, based in medical schools and hospitals," which attempted to exert hegemony in the guise of "scientific medicine" over other medical systems (1975:581). In addition to the competition posed by heterodox practitioners, elite regular physicians faced considerable competition within their own ranks. Because of the proliferation of proprietary medical schools after the Civil War, individuals of relatively humble origins could become regular physicians following several months to a year or two of medical education. Graduates of more prestigious medical schools objected to this situation. During the late nineteenth century, these elite regular physicians voiced increasing concern about the quality of medical education, particularly in the proprietary schools, and about competition from the ever growing number of physicians, both regular and heterodox. They felt that regular physicians with less prestigious credentials than their own provided inferior health care and also saturated the medical marketplace, thus depressing physician earnings (Numbers 1997:231).

The AMA began to take on these concerns after undergoing a constitutional reorganization in 1901 that strengthened it nationally. In 1906, its Council on Medical Education, which had been formed two years earlier, conducted a survey of medical colleges. Of the 160 schools inspected, the council rated 82 as class A, 46 as class B, and 32 as class C. The report had significant consequences:

> Fifty schools agreed to require one year each of college physics, chemistry, biology, and a modern language before admission to the medical program. Sensing doom, a number of schools consolidated with other medical schools in their cities, combining facilities and staffs. Other schools realized that they did not have the resources to survive the heightened competition. By 1910 the number of schools had fallen from a high of 166 to 131. (Brown 1979:140)

At about the same time, elite physicians turned to corporate-sponsored foundations in their effort to gain ascendancy over regular physicians of humbler social origins and over rival medical systems, particularly homeopathy, eclecticism, and osteopathy. The direction that medical care, medical education, and medical research took in America in the twentieth century was largely shaped by philanthropic organizations sponsored by John D. Rocke-feller, including the General Education Board—which was guided by men such Frederick T. Gates, Henry S. Pritchett, and Abraham and Simon S. Flexner—and to a lesser degree by the Carnegie Foundation. The founda-tions exerted their influence primarily by sponsoring evaluations of medical education (especially the influential Flexner Report, discussed below) and by funding medical research (Brown 1979:111–34). Nearly half of the phil-anthropic foundation support to higher education between 1902 and 1934 went specifically to biomedicine. Gates, a Baptist minister who took charge of Rockefeller's philanthropic affairs in 1891, was a corporate liberal who re-garded medicine as a means of improving functional health and ameliorating class conflict (Berliner 1982:188). Inspired by William Osler's *Principles and Practice of Medicine,* Gates concluded that a "scientific" brand of medicine, based on research, would transcend the sectarian rivalries among allopaths, homeopaths, and other medical practitioners of the period. Despite John D. Rockefeller's predilection for homeopathy, Gates managed to convince him to sponsor the creation of the Rockefeller Institute for Medical Research in 1901, apparently on the basis of its public relations value. In his close asso-ciation with John D. Rockefeller, Jr., Gates functioned as part of the newly emerging managerial stratum that helped to make the transition from the robber-baron, rugged individualistic capitalism of the older Rockefeller to the more rationalized corporate capitalism of the younger Rockefeller (Brown 1979:41–43).

The Rockefeller Institute served as a model for "scientific" research based on the germ theory. According to Berliner, "while germ theory was a major progressive step in the development of medicine, scientists of the time exag-gerated the importance of specific etiology and neglected all that had been previously learned about the non-bacterial (e.g., social, environmental) fac-tors in disease causation and spread" (1985:81). Based on the observation of discrete pathogens under the microscope, germ theory, while certainly not a conscious creation of the capitalist class, served its interests well by allowing an emphasis on specific cures for specific diseases along with a corresponding neglect of the social origins of disease.

In recognizing that alternative medical systems, including non-Western ones, may also be scientific in that they engage in the systematic search for cause-and-effect relationships, many medical anthropologists have come to refer to the dominant medical paradigm in Western societies as "biomedi-cine" rather than "scientific medicine." According to Hahn and Kleinman, biomedicine exhibits a "primary focus on human pathology, or more accu-rately on physiology, even pathophysiology" (1983:306). As Brown asserts, the regular medical profession "discovered an ideology that was compatible with the world view of, and politically and economically useful to, the capitalist or corporate class and the emerging managerial and professional stratum" (1979: 171). It is notable that the new mode of medical production focused on pathogens as the cause of disease at a time when there was increasing labor unrest in the cities, populist sentiments were widespread among farmers and small-town people, and social medicine had recognized that many new illnesses had occupational and environmental underpinnings.

The emerging alliance around the beginning of the twentieth century between the AMA, which now consisted primarily of elite practitioners and medical researchers based in prestigious universities, and the industrial capitalist class ultimately permitted biomedicine to establish political and ideological dominance over rival medical systems. The state was a crucial third ally in this process. In capitalist societies, the state serves the interests of the dominant class by mediating class, racial/ethnic, and gender conflict in order to stabilize the system. According to Willis (1983:23), the dominance of biomedicine rests on an alliance between medical practitioners and the state, which in turn represents the interests of the corporate class.

The concept of "hegemony" is useful for understanding how the corporate class indirectly came to influence medical theory and practice. Antonio Gramsci developed this concept in the *Prison Notebooks* ([1929–1935] 1971), elaborating upon Marx and Engels's contention that the "ideas of the ruling class are in every epoch the ruling ideas" (Marx 1978:192). Hegemony refers to the process by which one class comes to dominate the cognitive and intellectual life of a society through structural rather than coercive means. This dominance is achieved through the diffusion of certain values, attitudes, beliefs, social norms, and legal precepts that, to a greater or lesser degree, come to permeate civil society. The worldview of the dominant group or ruling class is so thoroughly diffused and entrenched that it becomes the "common-sense" view of the entire society. The arenas of ideological-cultural transmission are numerous. Ruling classes utilize all institutionalized mechanisms through which perceptions are shaped—the mass media, schools, churches, conventional political parties, the family, and even medicine—to mold the beliefs, attitudes, and behavior of the masses. This process is not necessarily carried out with a conscious intention of shaping social thinking but results from the firm sense among elites that their ideas are superior to those of others. For example, the idea that people are responsible for their own successes and failures (a notion that is contradicted in the daily experience of poor and working-class individuals) is heavily promoted in society because the successful believe it to be true. The effect, however, is (to some degree) to keep poor and working-class people from questioning blatant social inequalities that make success much easier for some than for others (Femia 1981; Bocock 1986).

In this book, I use the term medical hegemony to refer to the process by

34

which capitalist premises, concepts, and ideology influence biomedical diagnosis and therapy (Waitzkin 1983:139–41). This process is evident in the way
regular physicians embraced the germ theory, which "emphasizes discrete,
specific, and external causal agents of disease" (Brown 1979:75) and virtually
ignored the broader environmental conditions that contribute to it: biomedicine focuses on the individual and diverts attention from the social and economic causes of disease. According to Navarro, the corporate class came to
support this version of medicine, in which

> disease was not an outcome of specific power relations but rather a biological
> individual phenomenon where the cause of disease was the immediately observ-
> able factor, the bacteria. In this redefinition, clinical medicine became the branch
> of scientific medicine to study the biological individual phenomena and social
> medicine became that other branch of medicine which would study the distribu-
> tion of disease as the aggregate of individual phenomenon. Both branches shared
> the vision of disease as an alteration, a pathological change in the human body
> (perceived as a machine), caused by an outside agent (unicausality) or several
> agents (multicausality). (1986:166)

Physician-patient interactions frequently reinforce hierarchical structures
in the larger society by focusing on the need for the patient to comply with
a social superior's or expert's judgment. In treating a patient experiencing
job-related stress that manifests itself in diffuse symptoms, for example, the
physician may prescribe a sedative to calm the patient or to help him or
her cope with an onerous work environment rather than challenging the
power of the patient's employer or supervisor. In the United States, biomedicine incorporates core values, metaphors, beliefs, and attitudes such as
self-reliance, rugged individualism, independence, pragmatism, empiricism,
atomism, militarism, and a mechanistic concept of the body and its "repair,"
all of which are communicated to patients (Stein 1990:63–70). The values of
American biomedicine are undoubtedly rooted in the "frontier mentality" as
that developed within a capitalist worldview.

Through its alliance with corporations and the state, the medical establishment was able to carry out reforms that solidified its hegemony. One important step involved changes in licensing laws around the turn of the century.
As a result of their ties with state legislatures, physicians affiliated with the
AMA were able to gain dominance over licensing boards when new licensing laws started to be passed in the 1890s. According to Berliner, the AMA's
decision to grant licensure only to graduates of schools deemed acceptable
by the American Council of Medical Education in 1906 "proved to be the
beginning of the end of the pluralistic system of medical care in the United
States" (1975:583). The AMA was able to further limit the supply of medical
graduates to those of the "scientific" schools by designing the licensing ex-

aminations in such a way that graduates from these schools would fare better than graduates of other schools.

The hegemony of biomedicine was further advanced as a result of the Flexner Report of 1910, which was sponsored by the corporate-based Carnegie Foundation following the AMA's recommendation that a comprehensive survey of the quality of medical education be made. Abraham Flexner, a businessman, wrote the report based upon his visits to regular, homeopathic, eclectic, and osteopathic schools in the United States and Canada. While the Flexner Report may have contributed in some ways to improving the quality of medical education in the United States, it also had other important effects on the American medical system, including the following:

(1) It was a factor in the rapid decline in the number of biomedical schools — from 162 in 1906 to 95 in 1916 and 79 in 1924 — and in the number of regular physicians per 100,000 population — from 173 in 1900 to 137 in 1920 and 125 in 1930 (Ehrenreich and Ehrenreich 1978:56).

(2) It contributed to the drastic change in socioeconomic, ethnic, and gender composition of the regular medical profession. Before the Flexner Report, access to a medical career was relatively open; afterwards it was largely confined to those of the upper and upper-middle classes. In 1910 there were eight medical schools that catered to African Americans as well as a substantial number that primarily served women; the Flexner Report contributed to the closing of all but two of the black medical schools — the one at Howard University in Washington, D.C., and Meharry Medical College in Nashville, Tennessee — and all but one of the women's medical schools (Ehrenreich and Ehrenreich 1978:64).

(3) It indirectly pushed heterodox medical schools, particularly osteopathic but also chiropractic ones to some extent, to orient their curricula to those of the biomedical schools.

(4) It contributed to the creation of a medical paradigm that views the body as a series of parts that can be repaired or replaced.

Osherson and AmaraSingham contend that the Flexner Report contributed to the mechanical view of the body by strongly emphasizing "(1) *the parts-of-a-whole curriculum;* (2) *a reductionist approach* to the human body; (3) *the central role of instrumentation* in diagnosis and therapy, and subspecialization of the physician; and (4) an emphasis on *efficacy and standardization,* with relative inattention to the social context of treatment" (1981:227). In essence, the new biomedical model discarded the view of the human body as an integrated organism in which effects on one part of the body influence the rest of body and ignored the advances made in social medicine by Rudolf Virchow and others during the late nineteenth century. As Stark observes, "modern allopathic or 'post-Flexnerian' medicine was less the outgrowth of earlier struggles against disease than an alternative to such Popular Health

36

Movements as Thomsonianism (in the U.S.) and to populist advocacy of social reform as the best medicine" (1982:429).

In large part, the Flexner Report represented a culmination of processes that regular medical reformers had initiated a few decades earlier. These reformers had come to favor a medical paradigm that was compatible with capitalist interests—a convergence that ironically was often more readily recognized by corporate managers such as Frederick Gates than by capitalist industrialists such as John D. Rockefeller, Sr., and Andrew Carnegie. One does not have to subscribe to a simplistic conspiracy theory that capitalist industrialists foisted the biomedical paradigm upon an unwitting regular medical profession seeking legitimation and improved socioeconomic status. Relationships between the biomedical profession and the corporate-sponsored foundations were complex (Hess 1997:58–67). For example, biomedical leaders like Simon Flexner and William Welch, a well-known medical scientist and the first dean of Johns Hopkins Medical School, guided the "funding tastes of Rockefeller, Jr., and Gates, who in turn influenced the largesse of Rockefeller, Sr." (Hess 1997:62–63).

The decision of the corporate-sponsored philanthropies, particularly the Rockefeller Foundation, to fund only the regular medical schools defined as superior (grade A) by the Flexner Report, and also to deny funding to the heterodox medical schools in part contributed to the demise of homeopathy and eclecticism (Rothstein 1972:298–325). Corporate-sponsored foundations were willing to fund only biomedical schools that conducted supposedly nonsectarian, "scientific" research in elaborate laboratories. The findings of the Flexner and AMA evaluations of medical schools prompted state examining boards not to test graduates of low-rating schools. As Brown aptly argues, "The Flexner report united the interests of elite practitioners, scientific medical faculty, and the wealthy capitalist class" (1979:155).

Following the Flexner Report, organized biomedicine continued to use licensure as a mechanism to attain dominance. Indeed, Flexner regarded state licensing boards as vehicles of medical reform. Rhetorically, licensure aims at ensuring that graduates of biomedical schools are qualified to practice. In reality, licensure is a multi-faceted and even contradictory process that organized biomedicine has utilized in its effort to contain those heterodox medical systems that attempted to professionalize. As Willis observes,

> The medical profession gains state patronage through being 'allowed' a monopoly of occupationally generated definitions of service . . . . [Medicine] mediates the relation between individuals and their bodies, and the state. However medicine is not only a mechanism of reproduction but also a beneficiary. The major benefit, which flows from its alliance with the dominant class, . . . is medical dominance. (1983:16)

Licensure functions as a gate-keeping mechanism that protects health practitioners from competition. It defines the boundaries of legitimate practice, educational criteria, and rates of admission.

Heterodox medical groups have attempted to use licensure as a way to achieve legitimation in the larger society while restricting purportedly less-qualified practitioners within their own ranks. When these groups conflict with biomedicine during this process, the state tends to side with the latter; however it does, at times, respond to the demands of heterodox or alternative practitioners (Gevitz 1988a:37). But while the state may make concessions to professionalizing heterodox medical systems and their sponsors, it does not do so in a way that directly challenges either capitalist ideology or the role of biomedicine in sustaining that ideology. The state must simultaneously maintain or improve the process of capital accumulation, including within the health sector, and create a sense of entitlement on the part of the general public. When heterodox medical systems are granted partial legitimacy, they often undergo a subtle co-optative process as they incorporate aspects of the biomedical model and thereby inadvertently contribute to biomedical dominance.

In addition to licensing, the institution of examinations helped to restrict heterodox practitioners. Beginning in the 1920s, American biomedical groups in various states lobbied for the passage of laws requiring basic science examinations whose content closely resembled that of biomedical board examinations. Initially these examinations, which followed biomedical premises, barred many graduates of heterodox medical schools from practicing. According to Gevitz,

> All in all, from 1927 through 1932, of 3697 M.D.s examined by the seven basic science boards, 3313 (89.6%) passed. Of 229 D.O.'s 145 (63.%) did so, and of 135 chiropractors, 36 (26.6%) received certificates. (1988a:48)

By 1942 17 states had implemented basic science examinations that forced heterodox medical schools, particularly the osteopathic and chiropractic ones, to orient their curricula to more closely correspond to those in the biomedical schools. When the graduates of the osteopathic and chiropractic schools began to achieve high pass rates on the basic science examinations, the examinations were dropped because they no longer fulfilled their original purpose. Ironically, the examinations were also barring a significant number of M.D.s from practicing—a factor that also prompted organized biomedicine to alter its position on them.

In essence, American medicine after the turn of the century underwent a transformation from a relatively pluralistic form to a dominative one. In the last decades of the nineteenth century, as Brown notes, "with the convergence in practice and education of homeopaths, eclectics, and regular physicians, it was possible to assure the dominance of scientific training and politically necessary to ignore, for the moment, sectarian separations" (1979:89). Eventually, however, a reductionist scientific paradigm compatible with the worldview of the corporate class made it possible for biomedical physicians to gain solid dominance over what they sometimes referred to as "irregular" practitioners. Heterodox medical systems that had a somewhat more holistic view of health and disease found themselves at a disadvantage and responded by adopting the theory and practice of the biomedical physicians. Riska maintains that "by 1930, allopathic medicine had managed to eliminate the pluralistic character of American medicine: there were few remaining traces of sectarian medicine and of the self-care movement" (1985:31).

THE DEMISE OF TWO PROFESSIONALIZED HETERODOX MEDICAL SYSTEMS: HOMEOPATHY AND ECLECTICISM

As biomedicine gained dominance, homeopathy and eclecticism died out. The practice and education of homeopaths, eclectics, and regular physicians converged, partly as a result of the new licensing laws. In 1903 the AMA eliminated its ban on homeopathic and eclectic physicians so long as they did not designate themselves as such (Brown 1979:89). In this way, the diminishing ranks of the homeopathic and eclectic physicians were combined in a united effort with the AMA to counteract the growing popularity of new heterodox practitioners, particularly osteopaths but also chiropractors and naturopaths. The AMA also formed an alliance with the pharmaceutical industry— in keeping with its emphasis on the administration of drugs—to mount a concerted campaign against homeopathy in the 1890s and 1900s (Coulter 1973). Furthermore, the pharmaceutical industry indirectly supported regular medicine by placing numerous advertisements in its journals (Starr 1982: 134).

Another factor in the decline of homeopathy was that homeopaths' belief that disease could be best treated by administering small dosages of drugs and by altering environmental conditions was incompatible with the reductionist perspective of biomedicine with its emphasis on high doses of medication. After the turn of the century, most homeopathic physicians resigned themselves to absorption into biomedicine.

The combination of lack of funding and new licensing requirements hurt homeopathic medical schools. Corporate-sponsored foundations preferred to fund "scientific" medical schools. Following the development of unified examining boards, according to Kaufman, homeopathic courses were relegated to a minor role in the curriculum. The instruction in homeopathy was given short shrift in favor of the subjects required for licensure. Obviously, the homeopathic colleges could not compete with colleges having large endowments and enough resources to pay high salaries and purchase the latest instruments. (1971:175)

As a result, many homeopathic schools either closed or converted themselves into biomedical schools. The number of homeopathic schools declined from 22 in 1900 to 12 in 1910 and 5 in 1920 (Rothstein 1972:287). Only two homeopathic colleges, the New York Homeopathic College and the Hahnemann Medical College (both of which were granted class A ratings by the AMA), remained in existence in 1923. In 1936, the New York Homeopathic College transformed itself into the New York Medical College (Kaufman 1971:178). Hahnemann Medical College decreased its course offerings in homeopathy in 1936 but granted the "Doctor of Homeopathic Medicine" until the late 1940s (Rothstein 1972:297). It eliminated its required homeopathic courses in the early 1950s and taught its last elective course in homeopathy in the early 1960s. Hahnemann Medical College today retains the name of the founder of homeopathy but functions as a biomedical institution in the fullest sense of the word.

Organized homeopathy managed to linger on until the mid-twentieth century. The International Hahnemannian Association discontinued publishing its proceedings in 1947, and it ceased to exist in 1957 when its few remaining members joined the AIH (Coulter 1973:450). Fourteen "high potency" practitioners had formed the American Foundation for Homeopathy (AFH) in 1921 in a desperate attempt to curtail the complete demise of American homeopathy. Although the foundation's postgraduate course was offered into the 1960s, it trained only small numbers of physicians in homeopathy. Fewer than 150 physicians, many of them foreigners who did not intend to practice in the United States, took the course over a period more than 40 years (Kaufman 1971:173–74). Furthermore, the AIH refused to cooperate with the AFH. Various other heterodox practitioners, however, have exhibited an ongoing interest in homeopathy. For example, several chiropractors created "homeopathic colleges" in the 1950s (Kaufman 1971:182).

More or less at the same time as homeopathic schools were becoming biomedical schools or shutting their doors, the eclectic schools were also undergoing a decline. In 1902 there were eight eclectic medical schools, one each in Cincinnati, New York, Lincoln (Nebraska), San Francisco, St. Louis, Atlanta, and Indianapolis, and two in Chicago (Haller 1994:214). Two of these schools had closed their doors by 1910 and four others had done so by 1915 (Burrow 1963:87). In 1935, the American Association of Medical Colleges refused to recognize the Eclectic Medical School, the last of the eclectic schools, because it allegedly had an inappropriate board of trustees, insufficient hospital and clinical facilities, and lack of research. This Mecca of eclecticism offered its final course in 1938–39 (Coulter 1973:93).

The National Eclectic Medical Association actually continued to exist until the 1960s. Haller notes that the "last record of the association and its quarterly journal was the September-December issue in 1965, which noted the coming 1966 convention for June 15–17" in Hot Springs, Arkansas (1994:247). A relatively recent effort to rejuvenate eclecticism occurred in 1982 when two naturopathic physicians established the Eclectic Institute Incorporated, a botanical research enterprise situated at the National College of Naturopathic Medicine in Portland, Oregon (Haller 1994:247).

A MODEL OF THE AMERICAN
DOMINATIVE MEDICAL SYSTEM

Navarro contends that the class structure of American society is "reflected in the composition of the different elements that participate in the health sector, either as owners, controllers, or producers of services" (1976:138). Members of the upper class and, to a lesser degree, the upper-middle class predominate on the boards of foundations involved in health policy decision-making, private and state medical schools, and voluntary hospitals. The remaining social classes are distributed in positions of differential power within the biomedical division of labor. Most regular physicians are white upper-middle-class males. Paraprofessionals (e.g., nurses, physical and occupational therapists, technologists, and technicians) fall into the lower-middle class. Most of them are female and about nine percent are African American. Finally, "the working class per se of the health sector, the auxiliary, ancillary, and service personnel represent 54.2 percent of the labor force, who are predominantly women (84.1 percent) and who include an overrepresentation of blacks (30 percent)" (Navarro 1976:138).

As a result of affirmative action policies and other factors, such as the declining prestige of biomedicine as a career, the percentage of female M.D.s in the United States had risen to 18.8 percent by 1993 (Weiss and Lonnquist 1997:159–60). Whereas women constituted 28.9 percent of first-year biomedical students in 1980, they constituted 42.2 percent in the mid-1990s (Weitz 1996:241). Despite significant inroads into the corridors of biomedicine and the creation of the American Medical Women's Association, however, female physicians essentially function as second-class citizens within their profession and confront a "glass ceiling" on their upward mobility. Female physicians tend to be concentrated in the less prestigious specialities, such as family practice, pediatrics, and psychiatry. They are more likely to be

41

salaried employees than are male physicians, are underrepresented as medical educators and researchers, and generally do not supervise large, prestigious health facilities, teaching hospitals, or large medical centers (Lorber 1993:63). The growing proportion of female physicians has occurred in conjunction with the growing bureaucratization and routinization of biomedical practice in the United States and elsewhere (Riska and Wegar 1993:80–81).

Affirmative action policies have also contributed to an increased presence of members of various ethnic minorities in the biomedical profession. Although ethnic minorities constituted about one-quarter of the population of the United States in the mid-1990s, they made up almost one-third of first-year medical students (Weitz 1996:241–42). However, Asian Americans/Pacific Islanders comprised 15.6 percent of these first-year medical students, whereas African Americans (8.6 percent), Native Americans (0.8 percent), Mexican Americans (2.6 percent), and Puerto Ricans (1.9 percent) were still disproportionally underrepresented.

Navarro's description of the American health sector refers primarily or exclusively to its biomedical component, but the American medical system as a whole, including heterodox medical subsystems (which I generally refer to as "systems" for purposes of simplification) also tends to replicate class, racial/ethnic, and gender divisions in the larger society. While to a certain degree the multiple systems that existed during the nineteenth century reflected these social divisions as well, the correlation was not as strong. Regular physicians at the time were drawn from a wider spectrum of social classes then they were during the twentieth century, and most homeopathic physicians enjoyed a higher socio-economic status than did the great bulk of their regular counterparts. Figure 1 illustrates in rank order the major components of the dominative medical system that became entrenched in American society over the course of the twentieth century.

The biomedical establishment attempts to control the production of health care specialists, define their knowledge base, dominate the medical division of labor, eliminate or narrowly restrict the practices of heterodox or alternative practitioners, and deny laypeople and alternative healers access to medical technology. As we have seen, biomedicine achieved scientific superiority and clearly established hegemony over heterodox medical systems in large part because of financial backing for its research activities and educational institutions, first from corporate-sponsored foundations and later from the federal government. Ultimately, the ability of biomedicine to achieve dominance depends on support from the "strategic elite." Freidson maintains:

> A profession attains and maintains its position by virtue of the protection and patronage of some strategic elite segment of society which has been persuaded that there is some special value in its work. Its position is thus secured by the political

Figure 1   The American Dominative Medical System

Biomedicine
Osteopathic Medicine (a parallel medical system focusing on primary care)
Professionalized Heterodox Medical Systems
    Chiropractic
    Naturopathy
    Acupuncture
Partially Professionalized or Lay Heterodox Medical Systems
    Homeopathy
    Herbalism
    Bodywork
    Body/Mind Medicine
    Midwifery
Anglo-American Religious Healing Systems
    Spiritualism
    Seventh-day Adventism
    New Thought Healing Systems (Christian Science, Unity, Religious Science, etc.)
    Pentecostalism
    Scientology
Folk Medical Systems
    European American Folk Medicine
    African American Folk Medicine
    Vodun
    Curanderismo
    Espiritismo
    Santeria
    Chinese American Folk Medicine
    Japanese American Folk Medicine
    Hmong American Folk Medicine
    Native American Healing Traditions

and economic influence of the elite which sponsors it—an influence that drives competing occupations out of the same area of work, that discourages others by virtue of the competitive advantages conferred on the chosen occupation and that requires still others to be subordinated to the profession. (1970:72–73)

The unspecified strategic elite that Freidson refers to includes members of the corporate class interested in health issues, their political allies in the executive and legislative branches of the federal government, and health policy makers in both the government and private foundations and think tanks.

Nevertheless, biomedicine's dominance over rival medical systems has never been absolute. The state, which primarily serves the interests of the corporate class, must periodically make concessions to subordinate social groups in the interests of maintaining social order and the capitalist mode of production. As a result, certain heterodox practitioners, with the backing of affluent clients and particularly influential patrons, were able to obtain legitimation in the form of full practice rights (e.g., osteopathic physicians who may pre-

43

scribe drugs and perform the same procedures as biomedical physicians) or limited practice rights (e.g., chiropractors, naturopaths, and acupuncturists). Alternative medical systems of various sorts continue to function and even thrive in both rural and urban areas. Biomedicine is unable to establish complete hegemony in part because elites permit other forms of therapy to exist, but also because patients seek the services of alternative healers for a variety of reasons, such as the bureaucratic and iatrogenic drawbacks of biomedicine as well as its therapeutic limitations. Lower social classes, racial and ethnic minorities, and women have often utilized alternative medicine as a forum for challenging not only biomedical dominance but also, to a degree, the hegemony of the corporate class in the United States. Members of these social categories have often found that folk and religious healers tend to provide them with more culturally meaningful, personal, and holistic health care than biomedical and other professional practitioners generally do.

Alternative medicine under the umbrella of the "holistic health movement" has made yet another strong comeback in the United States. This eclectic movement incorporates elements from Eastern medical systems, the human potential movement, and New Ageism, as well as earlier Western heterodox medical systems. A Harvard Medical School study in the early 1990s estimated that one-third of the population had used at least one alternative therapy in the previous year (Eisenberg et al. 1993). The researchers also found that patients paid about three-quarters of the almost $14 billion cost out-of-pocket because few insurance companies cover alternative care. In contrast, the annual out-of-pocket expenses for hospitalization were $12.8 billion. A follow-up of the Harvard study found a 47.3 percent increase in total visits to alternative therapists between 1990 and 1997, from 427 million to 629 million (Eisenberg et al. 1998). The study also indicated that "a significantly higher proportion of alternative therapy users saw an alternative practitioner in 1997 (46.3%, equivalent to 39 million people) than in 1990 (36.3%, equivalent to 22 million people)" (Eisenberg et al. 1998:1571).

As a result of its perceived contribution to functional health, which is essential for maintaining a productive workforce, entry into the role of health care provider in capitalist societies has historically been seen as a vehicle for improving one's socioeconomic status. When individuals from lower social strata are denied entrance into the dominant medical profession, they sometimes turn to alternative healing groups within biomedicine. Emerging health occupations such as nursing that seek to advance their interests may attempt one of two strategies: professionalization or unionization. Krause asserts:

> In general, professionalization appeals to a social consensus model: it aims to gain acceptance by all other occupational groups in the field and by the general public, of the new higher value of the striving occupation and the legitimacy of its

requests for more rewards, power, status, and so forth. Unionization, in contrast, is a conflict-based process: the individuals and the occupations band together to force from the power structure and the society what it will not give up without such a struggle. (1977:76)

Although health occupational groups (e.g., nurses, medical technologists and technicians, etc.) that find themselves subordinate to administrators and physicians in the biomedical division of labor occasionally adopt the unionization approach, almost invariably they adopt professionalization as a strategy of collective social mobility. Similarly, in nineteenth-century America, homeopathy, botanic medicine or eclecticism, and hydropathy embarked upon a drive for professionalization, as have osteopathy, chiropractic, naturopathy, and, most recently, acupuncture in the twentieth century. Professionalization, however, is a subtle but highly effective hegemonic process by which alternative practitioners internalize some, if not many, of the philosophical premises, therapeutic approaches, and organizational structures of biomedicine. As Larson observes, "the persistence of profession as a category of social practice suggests that the model constituted by the first movements of professionalization has become an ideology—not only an image which consciously obscures real social structures and relations" (1977:xviii). In a similar vein, Willis (1983:16) argues that the "ideology of professionalism" promotes ideological hegemony and thus support for corporate capitalism.

As professionalized heterodox medical systems, osteopathy, chiropractic, and, to a lesser degree, probably naturopathy held out the promise of improved social mobility to thousands of lower-middle- class and working-class individuals as well as members of other social categories. In attempting to enter the medical marketplace, as Larkin asserts, "innovatory groups in medical science often commence with low status, particularly through their involvement in activities [e.g., spinal manipulation] previously regarded as outside of a physician's or surgeon's role" (1983:5). As the new medical system grows, it accumulates

> more and more members who are interested in making a good living and in raising their status in the outer world. In the health sphere, this means that they become more concerned with obtaining respectable (or at least respectable-looking) credentials, providing services that more clearly follow the medical model, and eventually even developing relationships with the orthodox medical world. (Roth 1976:40–41)

In their effort to professionalize themselves, homeopathic physicians underwent this process and eventually were absorbed by organized biomedicine. In subsequent chapters, I explore the tensions that have occurred in other heterodox medical systems, particularly osteopathy, chiropractic, naturopathy, and acupuncture, between co-optation and/or absorption into biomedicine on the one hand and preservation of therapeutic and organizational distinctiveness on the other hand.

BIOMEDICINE AS THE DOMINATIVE ACTOR
IN THE AMERICAN MEDICAL SYSTEM

Biomedicine constitutes the predominant subsystem or "ethnomedicine" in American society—one that has been controlled and promoted primarily by upper- and upper-middle-class European Americans (Hahn and Kleinman 1983:306). Unlike various ethnomedical or folk systems found among particular racial and ethnic minorities and working-class people in the United States, biomedicine constitutes a professionalized system. Freidson (1970) has likened the position of biomedicine in modern societies to that of a state religion. But state religions as instruments of social control were always subordinate to the wishes of the ruling elites of their societies. As I explained in the introduction, the professional dominance of biomedicine is *delegated* rather than *absolute*. The corporate class and its political allies delegate power to biomedicine in the form of financial support and licensing. Larson views "professionalization" as a process aimed at monopoly: "monopoly of opportunities in a market of services or labor and, inseparably, monopoly of status and work privileges in an occupational hierarchy" (1979:609). She notes that professional privilege acts as a *petit bourgeois* endeavor that permits an occupational group to share in the profits that the capitalist class extracts from the working class. Because professions such as biomedicine and law are able to control the production of their own knowledge, they are able to translate the "accumulation of 'cultural property' or symbolic capital" into dominance over competing occupational groups, including alternative health practitioners (Larson 1979: 621). Competing occupational groups both within and outside of medicine (e.g., nurse practitioners, osteopathic physicians, chiropractors, lay midwives) that wish to professionalize, however, have often questioned biomedicine's claim to therapeutic exclusivity.

Although American biomedical physicians still exert a great deal of control over their work, some scholars have argued that they are undergoing a process of "deprofessionalization" or even "proletarianization." Haug (1975:197) argues that three forces may be contributing to this process: the computerization of diagnosis and prognosis; the emergence of new occupations, such as physicians' assistants and nurse practitioners, which have assumed many of the tasks carried out by the physician in the past; and a growing public awareness of health matters and an associated distrust of biomedicine's ability to address a wide variety of diseases, particularly chronic ones. In a somewhat different vein, Oppenheimer hypothesizes that in a number of professions, including biomedicine, "a white collar proletarian type of worker is now replacing the autonomous professional type of worker in the upper strata of professional-technical employment" (1973:213). McKinlay and Arches elaborate upon Oppenheimer's thesis by arguing that as a result of the bureaucratization that is being forced on medical practice by the logic of capitalist expansion, physicians are being "proletarianized," despite their still relatively high incomes. They assert that "physicians are being forced to relinquish control over the disposition of their own labor power, which assumes market commodity features and, as for most other workers in societies dominated by capitalism, is increasingly sold in exchange for wages and salaries and is involved in the creation of surplus value for some other party at an ever increasing rate of exploitation" (McKinlay and Arches 1985:171). Derber, however, rejects the thesis that biomedical physicians are being proletarianized. He maintains that physicians "have been drawn into a historically unique relation to providers of capital, conceptualized here as a special mode of 'sponsorship' in which their vulnerability to control has been significantly mitigated" (1983:561). Hospitals, the principal sponsors of physicians, have not been able to sever the relationship between physicians and patients, despite the fact that they often impose bureaucratic constraints that challenge biomedical autonomy.

In order to understand the dynamics behind the processes which Haug, Oppenheimer, McKinlay and Arches, and Derber observe, we must see how changes in the political economy shape the organization of American medical care. It was noted earlier that around the turn of the century, the AMA was an elitist group of physicians who were strongly interested in biomedical science. In 1913 the AMA expanded to include members belonging to state and local medical societies (Burrow 1963:49). After World War I, the private physicians for whom biomedicine constituted a type of cottage industry gained control of the AMA, which meant that many of the scientists who worked in medical schools, research laboratories, and teaching hospitals moved out of the AMA (Kelman 1971). Before World II, solo practitioners dominated American biomedicine, and the AMA served their entrepreneurial interests well. Berliner (1982) asserts that between 1900 and 1970 biomedicine functioned as an "industrial mode of production" carried out by competing practitioners who produced a commodity purchased by patients. Ehrenreich and Ehrenreich succinctly summarize the transition that took place in American biomedicine after World War II:

> The postwar period has seen a steep decline in the role of the solo practitioner, both in the delivery of medical care itself, and in the medical power structure. Just as at the turn of the century the small factory gave way to the vast corporation, so the tens of thousands of one-man medical entrepreneurs have ceded the field to medical institutions—hospitals, and medical schools. In 1969, less than

twenty-nine percent of the nation's health expenditures went to private practitioners of all types; thirty-eight percent went to hospitals alone, and more than
sixty percent went to all the panoply of institutionalized health services, from hospital and nursing homes to public health agencies and institutional-based health
education and research. (1970:30–31)

With these developments, the political clout of the AMA has been diffused
by various organizations of specialists. The house of biomedicine has been
split into two establishments: the AMA and the "hospital doctors"—those
physicians who are employees in high-prestige teaching hospitals, university
hospitals, government hospitals, research centers, and health corporations. In
other words, an increasing number of physicians are becoming salaried employees of massive medical empires under private or state control. Physicians
in medical schools and teaching hospitals increasingly came to oppose AMA
policies after 1970 by cooperating with the federal government on various
cost-containment regulations that did not affect their own interests as much
as those of physicians in private practice (Krause 1996:45). The percentage
of biomedical physicians in the AMA rose from 51 percent in 1912 to 73 percent in 1963, but then fell to 65 percent by 1970 and to less than 50 percent
by 1990. The AMA has also been losing its place on state licensing boards
and national accrediting boards of other health occupations, such as physical
therapy. The traditional autonomy of the AMA itself has been undermined
in part by its heavy dependence for income from advertising in its journal,
particularly by pharmaceutical companies.

Beginning in the early 1970s biomedicine began to evolve into a "monopoly
mode of production" under which an increasing number of physicians became
salaried employees rather than independent entrepreneurs (Berliner 1982:
172). American medicine evolved into a "big business" in which health care
was increasingly concentrated in large health care corporations and medical
centers (Waitzkin and Waterman 1974:35). Scholars began to see biomedicine as embedded within a "medical-industrial complex" (Wohl 1984).

At the same time, health services have become matters of public concern,
particularly to third-party payers such as industry, insurance companies, government and labor, but also to consumers who ultimately must bear the bur-
den of rising costs in this area. In order to define and evaluate the "health
crisis" in the United States, various commissions have been formed in the
past few decades and have made many recommendations for public policy.
Alford (1972:137) notes that "predominant in all of these commissions are
hospital administrators, hospital insurance executives, corporate executives
and bankers, medical school directors, and city and state public health administrators." A striking feature of these commissions is the relative absence
of physicians, especially those in private practice. Salmon (1985) argues that

a "class-conscious corporate directorship" has come to assume considerable power over health policy decision-making and cost containment in health care. Professional review organizations evaluate physicians' decisions regarding hospitalization and treatment, and diagnosis related groups (DRGs) pay for hospital stays based on a fixed amount for a diagnosis.

As noted earlier, the role of the state in advanced capitalist societies is to resolve the contradictions that develop in a market economy and to reduce social tensions that may threaten the stability of the social system. The state must be responsive both to the requirements of the economy and to the organized demands of the public. Although the state must cater to the latter to some extent, it never questions the logic of a corporate economy and a stratified social system. Studies by Mills (1956), Domhoff (1967, 1990), and others have documented the upper-class origins of the top members of the American state, particularly those in the executive branch of the federal government. Consequently, when the state promotes changes in public policy, they tend to be in harmony with the interests of the corporate sector. According to Salmon, "state subsidization of the present health-care providers is promoting greater inroads by large corporations to participate in the industrialization of health services" (1975:610). Approximately 30 percent of all hospitals in 1990 were profit-making enterprises. The penetration of capital into health care has become a highly contradictory process. As Krause succinctly observes,

> Capitalism itself is divided . . . between the few sectors that make money as costs rise—medical technology, drugs, hospital supply—and the majority, which suffer increases in health coverage costs. The state acts with the majority of capitalist sectors and is gradually restricting for-profit medicine. Doctors thriving as owners of for-profit settings are already beginning to lose their advantage as regulation tightens. (1996:48)

Despite the tendency toward growing monopolization and concentration in biomedicine, other medical subsystems persist and even thrive, although often under precarious conditions, within the context of the American dominative medical system.

49

3

Osteopathic Medicine as a Parallel Medical System

Although osteopathy was developed toward the end of the nineteenth century, it was not until the twentieth century that it became a professionalized heterodox medical system and then, later, a parallel medical system to biomedicine. By the 1930s, it had split into two branches, osteopathic medicine and surgery. It adapted to American society and the dominative medical system by filling the vacuum in primary care left when biomedicine evolved into a capital-intensive, urban-based, and increasingly specialized endeavor. Osteopaths, despite a concerted effort on the part of regular physicians to restrict and later absorb them, achieved full practice rights in all 50 states and the District of Columbia by the early 1970s. Osteopathy had become a comprehensive health care system with a strong emphasis on primary care. But, at the same time, the therapeutic practices that had originally distinguished it from regular medicine had become less and less important to the majority of practitioners.

THE PHILOSOPHICAL PREMISES, THERAPEUTIC SCOPE, AND SOCIAL ORGANIZATION OF OSTEOPATHY

The early history of American osteopathy witnessed vigorous debates between the "lesion osteopaths," or straights, who wished to remain true to the principles delineated by Andrew T. Still, and the "broad osteopaths," or mixers, who were open to incorporating elements from regular medicine as well as from medical systems such as naturopathy and electrotherapy (Gevitz 1982:61–66). Although Still never believed the germ theory, many of his followers did, and they accepted parts of the *materia medica* that the "Lightning Bonesetter" had so vehemently rejected. At roughly the same time that regular medicine was evolving into biomedicine, osteopathy began to accommodate itself to the theory and practice of its parent. Osteopathic surgery provides a prime example. Still had objected to surgery except as a means of

50

last resort. In 1902, the Committee of Education of the American Osteopathic Association issued a statement that relaxed that injunction:

> Surgery is very closely related to osteopathy. They are identical in basis, in point of view, and in principles of diagnosis. Therapeutically, they are components of each other. Osteopathic cases sometimes require a little surgery, while nearly all surgical operations would be profitably supplemented by osteopathic treatment. The profession owes it to its patrons to provide opportunity for necessary surgery under osteopathic auspices, and it owes it to itself that it shall be a complete system, prepared to meet all conditions of disease. (American Osteopathic Association 1902)

Gradually osteopathy adopted other allopathic practices, including the administration of drugs, vaccines, and antibiotics. According to Reed (1932:14–15), by the early 1930s the curricula of osteopathic colleges closely resembled those of biomedical schools. With time, most of the specialties found in biomedicine became part of the osteopathic profession. Doctors of Osteopathy (D.O.s) began to refer to themselves as osteopathic physicians rather than osteopaths and to their practice as osteopathic medicine (or surgery) rather than osteopathy.

Despite the fact that osteopathy has adopted many of the practices of biomedicine, it continues to subscribe to a different philosophy. The most obvious difference between the training process in osteopathic medical schools and in biomedical schools is the inclusion of osteopathic manipulation therapy (OMT) in the curricula of the former. In the early days of the American School of Osteopathy, Still taught few therapies other than OMT (Hoover 1963:32). In contrast, the emphasis placed on the instruction of OMT today is relatively small, although it varies from program to program. OMT is also receiving little attention from researchers. One osteopathic physician laments that the bulk of osteopathic journals "publish little that cannot be found in the myriad of allopathic journals" (Campbell 1979:17).

Several circumstances are responsible for the changes in osteopathy. In surgery, as a result of a number of factors—the dearth of osteopathic surgeons, the lack of surgical training facilities in osteopathic institutions, and restrictive state licensing laws especially before 1920—osteopathic students who wished to become surgeons often were encouraged by their professors to obtain an M.D. degree after acquiring a D.O. degree (Gevitz 1982:62–63). Ironically, one of the individuals who followed this course of action was George A. Still, the grand-nephew of the founder of osteopathy. In education, despite the AMA's attempt to prohibit M.D.s from teaching in osteopathic colleges, their faculties have generally included at least a few regular physicians with no apparent interest in osteopathy. While it is difficult to assess the impact that such instructors have had on osteopathic students, it seems likely that their presence was one more reason why osteopathy evolved into osteopathic medicine.

Very little systematic attention has been given to the similarities and differences between M.D.s and D.O.s in their practices. It appears that in the past, patients who sought the services of osteopaths were largely those with chronic problems related to the musculoskeletal system (Booth 1924:69). Many such patients now turn to chiropractors. Whereas manipulative therapy has remained a central mode of treatment within chiropractic, it has become increasingly peripheral within osteopathic medicine. One study found that of the 188 respondents to a questionnaire sent to 308 osteopathic general practitioners, 39 percent indicated that they did not use OMT at all in their practices (McConnell et al. 1976:103). Although apparently most D.O.s manipulate patients on occasion, some employ OMT extensively and become known, generally by word-of-mouth among patients or through physician referrals, as being particularly adept in the treatment of musculoskeletal disorders.

Despite the growing similarity of osteopaths to biomedical physicians, professional and educational institutions serve to keep them distinctive professions. In many ways, the American Osteopathic Association (AOA), which was established in 1897, functions as the principal voice of osteopathic medicine. It exerts its influence in part through an affiliated group, the American Association of Colleges of Osteopathic Medicine, which sets educational standards for osteopathic medical schools. A total of 37 osteopathic institutions existed in the United States before 1910. The first, the American School of Osteopathy, was established in 1892, and 17 more were founded between 1895 and 1900 (Albrecht and Levy 1982:174). Early osteopathic colleges included the National School of Osteopathy (est. 1895) in Baxter Springs, Kansas; the Pacific School of Osteopathy (est. 1896), situated over time in different locations in Southern California; the Northern Institute of Osteopathy (est. 1896) in Minneapolis; the Colorado College of Osteopathy (est. 1897); the Southern College of Osteopathy (est. 1898) in Franklin, Kentucky; and the Atlantic School of Osteopathy (est. 1898) in Wilkes Barre, Pennsylvania (Booth 1924:86–92). In 1915 the AOA required its accredited colleges to maintain a four-year course of study. It recognized only the osteopathic colleges in Boston, Chicago, Des Moines, Kansas City, Missouri, Kirksville, Los Angeles, and Philadelphia (Gevitz 1982:80). The Massachusetts College of Osteopathy closed its doors in 1940, making it the last osteopathic school to close until the early 1960s, when the osteopathic school in Los Angeles was converted into a biomedical one.

While many of the debates over the role of OMT occurred within the osteopathic colleges, they also played themselves out in disagreements among different professional associations. A fair degree of tension exists between the AOA and the American Academy of Osteopathy, an organization that many D.O.s view as a quasi-certifying board for those practitioners who place great stress upon manipulative techniques. The Academy, which originated at the 1938 AOA convention as the Osteopathic Manipulation Therapeutic and Clinical Research Association, stresses the concept of total health care with an emphasis on the neuromuscular-skeletal system and offers postgraduate training in OMT to osteopathic physicians (Barnes 1971). Whereas most osteopathic physicians view OMT as an adjunct to be applied in specific instances, Academy members see it as central; they feel that mainstream osteopathic medicine has to a large extent forsaken its therapeutic birthright. Because of its continuing affiliation with the AOA, however, the Academy in effect constitutes a "loyal opposition" within the osteopathic profession.

De-emphasizing OMT served as a strategy by which many osteopathic physicians tried to counter the opinion within the biomedical community that osteopathy constituted a medical sect or cult. Osteopathic medicine continues to find itself ranked below biomedicine, however, despite having achieved a considerable amount of legitimacy in the larger American society. The use of OMT, then, has not been solely responsible for this low status. One other reason is that many osteopathic physicians are primary-care practitioners, and primary care itself is at the bottom of the biomedical profession's hierarchy. Another important reason is that D.O.s have generally been drawn from lower strata in the American class system than have M.D.s. The same features of the medical education system that have produced this class difference have also contributed to American osteopathy's growing similarity to biomedicine.

Although initially osteopathy attracted regular physicians and other individuals who wanted to practice a heterodox form of therapy, eventually many, if not most, of those who entered the profession did not do so because they wanted to become osteopaths; they wanted to become physicians per se but found admission to biomedical schools closed to them for various structural reasons. Many osteopathic students, indeed, view osteopathy as a "back door into medicine." In his study of students at four of the six osteopathic schools that existed at the time, for example, New (1958, 1960) found that most had entered osteopathic medicine either as a second choice to biomedicine or by accident:

> Only 34 out of the 103 students interviewed had not applied to any medical schools. Forty-four students went directly into an osteopathic college after their undergraduate training. The remaining took a variety of avenues: to another undergraduate school, to a graduate school, to a medical school, or any combination of these. A good number of them were in some other type of profession (pharmacy or chiropractic). Thus, they have a positive need for the development of rationales to assure themselves that they have not entered medicine via the

back door, a common accusation directed toward osteopathic students by some lay people. (1958:420)

Another, more recent, study produced similar results. From questionnaires filled out by 61 of the 64 graduates of the 1975 class of the Michigan State University College of Osteopathic Medicine, Sharma and Dressel (1975) found that 75 percent had applied to at least one biomedical school. Only 15 percent, however, had been accepted at one or more of these schools.

Historically, admission requirements have been less stringent at osteopathic than at biomedical schools, even though the AOA has tried to raise them. The AOA Board of Trustees mandated in 1920 that each accredited college require a minimum of a high school diploma for admission, and some schools required as much as two years of college. Many schools, however, intentionally kept lower admission requirements in order to remain accessible to students from poor families. George Laughlin, who became president of the Kirksville College of Osteopathy in the 1920s,

> argued that requiring two years of prior college work was hurting the underprivileged since they could least afford the additional schooling. As many of the students who did not meet this requirement came from farms and small towns, the standard had the indirect effect of causing a decline in the percentage of recent M.D. graduates deciding to locate in sparsely populated areas. Without this requirement, D.O. schools could meet the needs of the economically disadvantaged student and help alleviate the growing rural physician shortage. As it turned out, Laughlin's views and predictions had merit, since the D.O.s traditionally are highly represented in rural areas, and historically D.O. students have come from less affluent backgrounds than their M.D. counterparts. (Gevitz 1992:87–88)

New's study showed that osteopathy was indeed more open to the less affluent in the 1950s. Osteopathic students were more likely to come from blue-collar families than were their biomedical counterparts (New 1960:181). Of those who indicated their father's occupations, "36 students reported that their father was in clerical or small business types of profession, 27 students mentioned farmer or blue-collar work as their father's profession, and 16 students' fathers were in professional work" (New 1960:90). For most of the students in New's sample, osteopathic medicine clearly provided a means of upward social mobility. Furthermore, New found that 18 of the students in his sample were Jewish. Osteopathic schools appear to have provided an alternative by which academically qualified Jewish students could become physicians during the period 1920–1960, when many biomedical schools maintained implicit or explicit quotas on the number of Jews admitted (Cohen 1983:111).

Ironically, while osteopathic medicine initially was relatively open to women, in later years the percentage of women declined more rapidly in osteopathic medical schools than in biomedical schools (Cohen 1983:113).

Cohen suggests three possible reasons for this decline: the increasingly demanding academic prerequisites for admission, the growth in osteopathic schools following the closing of regular medical schools in the post-Flexner era, and the osteopathic profession's belief that one strategy for improving its status was to reduce the number of "the most visibly marginal of its members, women" (1983:114).

THE RELATIONSHIP BETWEEN OSTEOPATHY AND BIOMEDICINE

The relationship between osteopathy and biomedicine went through two stages. In the first, organized biomedicine attempted either to eliminate or to restrict osteopaths' practice rights. When biomedicine failed to accomplish these goals, it embarked upon the second strategy, an attempt to co-opt osteopathic medicine.

ORGANIZED BIOMEDICINE'S STRATEGY TO ELIMINATE OR RESTRICT OSTEOPATHY

In addition to branding osteopaths "cultists" (Fishbein 1932; Reed 1932), organized biomedicine employed a variety of tactics to destroy or restrict the ability of D.O.s to practice, including refusing them hospital privileges, forbidding them to consult with M.D.s, and attempting to limit their recognition by the government.

The AMA Judicial Council ruled in 1923 that the board of any private hospital could refuse privileges of hospitality to "any practitioner regardless of his so-called school of practice" (American Medical Association 1959). This policy was later approved by the AMA House of Delegates in 1936. In 1929 the house of delegates opposed a new American Red Cross policy that permitted its nurses to attend osteopathic patients (Rayack 1969:243). Partly as a result of organized biomedicine's opposition to having D.O.s practice in biomedical hospitals, D.O.s had to accept privileges in lower quality institutions or to establish their own hospitals.

In 1938 the house of delegates went further and ruled that any professional relationship between M.D.s and D.O.s was taboo. M.D.s were forbidden to consult D.O.s, to give lectures in osteopathic colleges or addresses before osteopathic professional associations, or to teach in osteopathic colleges. The AMA used such policies to minimize competition from D.O.s:

> the policy that it was "unethical" for M.D.s to voluntarily associate with osteopaths meant that if a D.O. sent a patient to an M.D. specialist, no report would

55

be given to the referring osteopath; or, if a report was given, it would often be by telephone to avoid "ethical" problems. Moreover, the specialist was presumably free to try to retain the patient or, at minimum, to induce the patient to switch to an M.D. Patients of D.O.s were thus denied the advantages of consultation given to patients of M.D. general practitioners, thereby reducing the effectiveness of D.O. competition. . . . Osteopaths were also denied permission to attend AMA sponsored continuing education programs. (Blackstone 1977: 416–17)

In the 1920s, after it failed to convince legislatures to eliminate independent osteopathic boards, organized biomedicine lobbied for a test in the basic sciences to be administered before the actual licensing examination. The immediate result was a relatively low pass rate among osteopathic students compared to that among biomedical students (e.g., 88.3 percent for M.D.s and 54.5 percent for D.O.s in 1930). Over the next decade or so, however, the pass rates of osteopathic students improved to the point that they compared favorably to those of biomedical students. Since the basic science examinations focused on subjects typically included in the curricula of biomedical schools, they undoubtedly contributed to the growing tendency in osteopathic schools to de-emphasize instruction in osteopathic manipulation therapy and related areas.

Organized biomedicine also opposed government recognition of D.O.s in a number of areas, for example, by supporting limited licensure, which prohibited D.O.s from using certain drugs or performing surgery. As late as 1966, the State Medical Association of South Carolina opposed full practice rights for D.O.s (Blackstone 1977:411). During World War II, the AMA successfully blocked the appointment of D.O.s as medical officers (Crawford 1962). Even though Congress authorized the appointment of D.O.s as military officers in 1956, no such appointments were made until July 1966 because of organized biomedicine's dominance of military hospitals (Blackstone 1977:415). The AMA also opposed government financial support of osteopathy, such as aid for osteopathic colleges. Despite such strategies, organized biomedicine was unable to curb the gradual but steady process by which the osteopathic profession began to obtain practice rights.

ORGANIZED BIOMEDICINE'S STRATEGY
TO CO-OPT OSTEOPATHY

By the 1950s, it was clear that osteopathy was not being eliminated: D.O.s succeeded in gaining full practice rights in most states by the end of the decade, and they constituted a large proportion of general practitioners or family physicians in certain states. Beginning in the early 1950s, organized biomedicine began to shift its policy concerning osteopathy to one of co-optation. The first significant indicator of a shift in policy appeared in 1951 when the AMA

Board of Trustees appointed a committee (generally referred to as the "Cline Committee") to study the relationship between biomedicine and osteopathy and to confer with representatives of the AOA on this issue.

Based upon the information it had gathered, the Cline Committee recommended that the AMA House of Delegates drop the label "cultist healing" in reference to osteopathic medicine and that it declare the relationship between M.D.s and D.O.s to be a matter left to the discretion of state medical associations. The House of Delegates voted to defer action on the committee's recommendations until a survey on education in osteopathic colleges could be completed. In June 1955, although the majority of the committee members basically reiterated their earlier recommendations, the House of Delegates adopted the minority report of one dissenting member, which stated that "if and when the House of Delegates of the American Osteopathic Association may voluntarily abandon the commonly so-called osteopathic concept, with proper deletion of said 'osteopathic concept' from catalogues of their colleges, and may approach the Board of Trustees of the American Medical Association with a request for further discussion of the relations of osteopathy and medicine, then the said Trustees shall appoint another special committee for such discussion" (Americal Medical Association 1955:736).

While deliberations concerning the relations between organized biomedicine and organized osteopathic medicine were taking place at the national level of the AMA, some state societies acted independently on this matter. During the 1950s, the California Medical Association and the California Osteopathic Association discussed the possibility of merger, and in 1961 the former in essence absorbed the latter. The two organizations agreed to: (1) convert the Los Angeles College of Osteopathy into a biomedical college, (2) arrange for the converted medical school to issue M.D. degrees to California D.O.s who held an unlimited California license to practice medicine, (3) create a temporary body for the transformed D.O.s until "they became absorbed into the regular county medical societies," and (4) lobby to prevent future licensure of D.O.s and to terminate the authority of the Board of Osteopathic Examiners, which would regulate only the few remaining D.O.s (Blackstone 1977:418–19). As a result of the absorption, the Los Angeles College of Osteopathy became the University of California, Irvine, College of Medicine, and most of the osteopathic hospitals in the state were converted into biomedical ones.

About the same time as the merger in California, the AMA House of Delegates decreed that each state medical society could determine whether or not to accept D.O.s as professional equals: "the test should be: Does the individual doctor of osteopathy practice osteopathy or does he in fact practice a method of healing founded on a scientific basis" (Judicial Council to the AMA House of Delegates 1961:774). In December 1968 the AMA approved the proposed merger of biomedical and osteopathic schools, suggesting that the latter should be accredited if they met certain AMA requirements, and also opened up internships and residencies in biomedical settings to D.O.s (Blackstone 1977:423).

THE ORGANIZATIONAL REJUVENATION
OF OSTEOPATHIC MEDICINE

In the wake of the California merger, many contemporary observers believed that it was only a matter of time before organized biomedicine absorbed osteopathic medicine on a state-by-state basis. Over 50 years ago, Reed hinted that osteopathy would go the way of certain nineteenth-century medical sects:

> In point of numbers, the growth of osteopathy has practically stopped. The failure to grow is probably due for the most part to two things: chiropractic, and the evolution of osteopathy. With the coming of chiropractic and the progressive evolution of osteopathy, osteopaths lost to the chiropractors those patients who were attracted by the "cure-all" feature. As osteopathy approached medicine and took over its therapeutic agents, the osteopaths came into competition with doctors of medicine on the latter's ground. In this competition they could hardly fail to be at a disadvantage. (1932:29)

Although there has been considerable convergence between osteopathic medicine and biomedicine, however, various trends in osteopathy since the California absorption suggest that it will remain a separate organizational entity for some time to come. Regardless of how rank-and-file members of the osteopathic profession may have viewed the California merger, the general leadership of the AOA reacted with strong disapproval and alarm. The AOA, for example, revoked the charter of the California Osteopathic Association as soon as the impending merger with the state medical association became apparent. Contrary to the expectation of organized biomedicine that the other state osteopathic societies would follow the example of the California chapter, the merger served as a rallying cry for the osteopathic profession in its struggle for survival.

Despite some other attempts at merger, such as those in Pennsylvania and in the state of Washington, the osteopathic profession successfully prevented the dissolution of state societies outside of California (Citizens Committee on Education for Health Care 1967). After most California D.O.s became M.D.s, the leadership of the osteopathic profession fell to the association in Michigan, which had the most osteopathic physicians after California (Walsh 1972: 1085). In 1969, in response to the conversion of the Los Angeles College of

Osteopathy into a biomedical institution, Michigan D.O.s decided that they would like to found a new college in Pontiac, Michigan.

When the osteopathic profession in Michigan realized that it lacked the funds to support an osteopathic college on its own, it turned to the state legislature (Citizens Committee on Education for Health Care 1967). Partly because D.O.s had provided much of the primary care in Michigan since World War II, the legislature approved the annexation in January 1970 of the private osteopathic college (est. 1964) in Pontiac to Michigan State University. The College of Osteopathic Medicine at Michigan State University became the first state-sponsored osteopathic school to share many of its facilities with an allopathic college. This event signaled the beginning of an organizational rejuvenation of osteopathic medicine. Of the 14 additional osteopathic colleges established since that date, six are state-supported institutions (in Texas, Oklahoma, West Virginia, Ohio, New Jersey, and New York; see table 1).

As a result of this government support, the number of osteopathic colleges tripled after the late 1960s, and the number of graduates increased from 394 in 1965 to 1,484 in 1985 (Ward and Tomaras 1985:720). Some 37,000 osteopathic physicians made up about four percent of the total physician population in the United States in 1998, and about one-third of them accounted for about one-third of all the general and family practitioners. Kenneth P. Moritsaga, the head of the Federal Bureau of Manpower, referred to osteopathic medicine as "one of the major underpinnings of the national policy to provide for the nation's primary-care health services" (quoted in "The D.O." 1980:42). As explained below, the growth of osteopathic medicine in the past several decades has helped to fill the void in primary care created by the increasing specialization and geographical maldistribution of biomedical physicians.

Following the California absorption, osteopathy won a number of legal reversals in several states. A state law passed in California made it illegal for a hospital to deny privileges to physicians—either biomedical or osteopathic (Denbow 1977:21). The supreme court of the state of Washington ruled in 1967 that a "quickie" medical school, which was established by the Washington State Medical Society for the sole purpose of allowing osteopathic physicians to exchange their D.O. degrees for M.D. degrees, was illegal, thereby stemming the loss of osteopathic physicians to biomedicine (Blackstone 1977: 420–21).

As we saw in chapter 2, the ability of organized biomedicine to limit the scope of osteopathy and other alternative medical systems, such as chiropractic and naturopathy, has depended upon winning the sponsorship of certain strategic elites. Its inability to exert complete dominance in this way, however, is evident in the fact that by the early 1970s osteopathic medicine had obtained full practice rights in all 50 states and the District of Columbia and equal status with biomedicine in the eyes of the federal government.

Table 1   Osteopathic Colleges in the United States

School	Charter Year	Status
Kirksville College of Osteopathic Medicine, Kirksville, MO	1892	private
Philadelphia College of Osteopathic Medicine, Philadelphia, PA	1898	private
Chicago College of Osteopathic Medicine, Midwestern University, Chicago, IL	1900	private
University of Osteopathic Medicine and Health Sciences, Des Moines, IA	1905	private
Kansas City College of Osteopathic Medicine, Kansas City, MO	1916	private
Michigan State University College of Osteopathic Medicine, East Lansing, MI	1964	state
University of North Texas College of Osteopathic Medicine, Fort Worth, TX	1966	state
Oklahoma State University College of Osteopathic Medicine, Tulsa, OK	1972	state
West Virginia School of Osteopathic Medicine, Lewisburg, WV	1974	state
Ohio University College of Osteopathic Medicine, Athens, OH	1975	state
University of Medicine and Dentistry of New Jersey School of Osteopathic Medicine, Stratford, NJ	1976	state
University of New England College of Osteopathic Medicine, Biddeford, ME	1976	private
New York College of Osteopathic Medicine, Old Westbury, NY	1977	state
College of Osteopathic Medicine of the Pacific, Pomona, CA	1977	private
Nova Southeastern University College of Osteopathic Medicine, Fort Lauderdale, FL	1979	private
Lake Erie College of Osteopathic Medicine, Erie, PA	1992	private
Florida College of Osteopathic Medicine, Tarpon Springs, FL	1994	private
Arizona College of Osteopathic Medicine, Midwestern University, Glendale, AZ	1995	private
Pikeville College of Osteopathic Medicine, Pikeville, KY	1997°	private
Touro University College of Osteopathic Medicine, San Francisco, CA	1997°	private

° Date of first entering class

Osteopathy's success in the face of seemingly insurmountable odds has to do in part with the vigorous campaign of professionalization that osteopathic physicians have carried on since the 1890s. This strategy entailed a concerted effort to share the medical marketplace with biomedicine. By 1903 osteopathic physicians had secured limited practice rights in Vermont, Illinois, Ohio, and Virginia despite the opposition of regular physicians (Hildreth 1942). Because of its astute lobbying activities, the osteopathic profession eventually gained full practice rights throughout the United States (see table 2). Furthermore, as early as 1910, D.O.s were able to obtain separate osteopathic licensing boards in 17 states (Burrow 1963:60). Osteopathic medicine has tended to be stronger in states in which it has had its own licensing board, such as California (at least prior to the 1961 incident), Michigan, and Penn-

Table 2   Decades in Which States Granted D.O.s Full Practice Rights

Decade	States Granting Full Practice Rights
1901–09	California, Connecticut, Massachusetts, Michigan, Texas
1910–19	Colorado, New Hampshire, Oregon, Virginia, Washington, Wyoming
1920–29	District of Columbia, Florida, Hawaii, Maine, Nevada, Oklahoma, Utah, West Virginia
1930–39	Arizona, Delaware, New Jersey, New Mexico, Tennessee
1940–49	Indiana, Nebraska, New York, Ohio, Rhode Island, South Dakota, Vermont, Wisconsin
1950–59	Alabama, Illinois, Kansas, Kentucky, Missouri, Pennsylvania
1960–69	Alaska, Georgia, Idaho, Iowa, Maryland, Minnesota, North Carolina, North Dakota, South Carolina
1970–73	Arkansas, Louisiana, Mississippi, Montana

Source: Information provided to author by American Osteopathic Association

sylvania, than in those states, such as New York, Wisconsin, and Indiana, in which D.O.s are licensed by composite boards or boards consisting of only biomedical physicians.

National and state osteopathic organizations have been actively involved in influencing legislation. The AOA maintains an office in Washington, D.C., which attempts to assure that D.O.s are recognized in health bills that directly benefit the profession and that they are represented on committees affecting government health policy. Although the AOA cannot lobby directly because of its legal status as an educational and research association, its Washington office makes arrangements for D.O.s to be available for congressional committee hearings on relevant bills. Many state osteopathic associations, however, do hire D.O.s and laypersons to lobby for the passage of legislation favorable to the profession. In addition, the osteopathic profession maintains a "grassroots system" for gaining recognition. D.O.s are encouraged to speak with U.S. senators and representatives and state legislators for this purpose. In some states, such as Michigan, many legislators are osteopathic patients. In their early drive for licensure, D.O.s often actively sought to treat various legislators as a way of demonstrating the value of osteopathic medicine (Russell 1974).

Indeed, the support of prominent people and organizations has been central to osteopathy's success. Strategic elites who were osteopathic patients include Theodore Roosevelt, Dwight Eisenhower, Nelson Rockefeller, Stuart Symington, and Howard Hughes. Rockefeller's personal D.O. frequently commuted from his New York City office to treat not only the former vice president but also Richard Nixon, Henry Kissinger, and various White House aides. The Rockefellers donated over $1,500,000 to osteopathic research and education and to the Kirksville College of Osteopathic Medicine, and General Motors Corporation donated $625,000 to the large osteopathic hospital in Detroit (Gross 1966:457). Amon Carter, a prominent Texas business magnate, donated $100,000 in the 1940s for a new osteopathic hospital in Fort Worth. In some states, strong support for the osteopathic profession has come from labor unions (e.g., the United Auto Workers in Michigan and Missouri).

Osteopathy has become an increasingly important element of American medicine not only because of osteopathic physicians' involvement in legislative debates and their support from some influential people, but also as a result of the structural problems that have plagued the American health care system since World War II. Three of these problems, which emanate from the growth of capital-intensive medicine and medical specialization, have particularly influenced the evolution of osteopathy and chiropractic: the diminishing proportion of primary-care physicians, the geographical maldistribution of physicians, and rising health care costs.

Because of an increase in specialization, the number of general practitioners in the United States dropped from 90 per 100,000 population in 1931 to 37 per 100,000 in 1962 (Huntley 1972). By the 1960s, too, their geographical distribution had become severely skewed:

> The majority of states have a below-the-national average physician to population ratio, and within states gross maldistribution creates shortages of crisis proportions for many areas. In the Kenwood area of Chicago there are 5 physicians per 100,000 population, whereas in the state as a whole the ratio is 133 per 100,000. North Carolina has a ratio of 100 per 100,000, but most doctors practice in the prosperous cities, leaving parts of the state's poorer rural areas almost totally deprived of medical services. (Smith 1972:209)

Since the early 1960s, federal and state governments, private foundations, and organized biomedicine have responded to this situation in various ways. In 1963 Congress passed the Health Professions Educational Assistance Act, which provided matching funds for the construction of new medical schools in order to encourage the production of primary-care physicians. In response to public and governmental pressure, the AMA made family practice a specialty in 1969, in an attempt to entice a greater number of medical graduates into primary care by increasing its prestige. In 1970 the Carnegie Commission advocated an increase in the number of medical schools and called for a greater commitment to general practice—a marked contrast to the recommendations of the 1910 Flexner Report.

In addition to these efforts, both public and private institutions began to look to osteopaths to help supply the need for primary medical care. D.O.s had already begun replacing M.D.s in primary care as early as the 1940s, when the situation that Walsh describes here for Michigan was replicated in many other states, including California, Missouri, Iowa, Ohio, Texas, Oklahoma, and Maine:

> In World II osteopaths were not drafted into the military medical services and in the wartime doctor shortage D.O.'s in Michigan provided needed medical care and gained a broad measure of public acceptance. . . . Probably the strongest factor in the continued rise of the osteopaths after the war was that a majority of them were general practitioners, whereas increasing numbers of M.D.'s entered the specialities or migrated out of the shortage areas. (Walsh 1972:1087)

The osteopathic profession was far slower in specializing than was biomedicine because it developed its hospital system relatively late and had limited funds for its schools. In 1967–68 the percentage of practitioners in general practice was 29 percent for biomedical physicians and 90 percent for osteopathic physicians; by 1978, the percentage had dropped significantly, to 18 percent, for biomedical physicians, but remained high, at 88 percent, for osteopathic physicians (Albrecht and Levy 1982:191).

A breakthrough for the financially strapped osteopathic schools occurred in 1951 when the United States Public Health Service awarded them renewable teaching grants, previously designated exclusively for biomedical and dental schools (Gevitz 1982:85). The primary-care shortage led to increasing support for osteopathic education. State support began in 1955 with a grant from the Pennsylvania legislature to the Philadelphia College of Osteopathic Medicine. From fiscal year 1965 through 1976, the Chicago, Des Moines, Kirksville, and Philadelphia osteopathic colleges were granted $65.8 million from the Health Professions Educational Assistance Act of 1963, the Health Manpower Act of 1968, and the Comprehensive Manpower Training Act of 1971 (Gevitz 1982:130).

Both federal and state governments appropriated funds to train osteopathic physicians as one strategy to help solve the shortage and geographic maldistribution of primary-care physicians. The Michigan state legislature approved the annexation of the private osteopathic college in Pontiac to Michigan State University principally because a high percentage of D.O.s were primary-care practitioners. Two statistics concerning D.O.s in Oklahoma, that more than three-fourths of them were general practitioners and that more than one half of these practiced in towns of fewer than 50,000, were of crucial importance in persuading the state legislature to establish a state osteopathic school (Jones 1978:27). An increased reliance on osteopathic physicians also seemed to be a way to address the problem of rising health care costs: legislators in several states were impressed that osteopathic physicians "earn about 25 percent less than traditional doctors in general practice and 15 percent less in specialty work" (Albrecht and Levy 1982:191).

Despite the traditional hostility of organized biomedicine to osteopathic medicine (and chiropractic), strategic elites in both the corporate and governmental sectors have come to regard D.O.s (and chiropractors) as health practitioners who can meet some of the primary-care needs of the larger society. Krause observes that:

> These two thriving branches of medical practice, whether or not they are accepted by the medical profession, are groups with their own hospitals and clinics, and are critically important in filling some of the gaps in community care. The shortage of physicians in medium-sized and small towns and in rural areas, for example, has left the field wide open to these two groups. Finally, in some regions of the nation, especially in parts of rural New England, the Middle West, and California, *they* and not the physicians constitute the top group, occupying the politically dominant "physician" role in local community politics and in the health service organization. Inside these settings, they order around the nurses and technicians precisely as do physicians in other towns. (1977:44–45)

The increasing public support for osteopathic medical schools, however, has had little to do with the osteopathic profession's claim to offer a distinct alternative to biomedicine. While to a greater or lesser extent many D.O.s stress the unique aspects of their approach to health care, especially in the treatment of musculoskeletal disorders, organized osteopathic medicine has tended to emphasize the notion that the quality of care it offers to the public is comparable, albeit in some ways superior, to that offered by biomedicine.

In part, the professionalization of osteopathic medicine and its legitimation as a parallel medical system since the late 1960s is related to the deprofessionalization of biomedicine. In a sense, osteopathic physicians gained professional prestige by default—that is, as a result of biomedicine's strong emphasis on the training of specialists, particularly in the period since World War II. While no direct evidence exists on the extent to which organized biomedicine was aware that D.O.s were filling a vacuum left by M.D.s, this phenomenon may have been a major factor in its attempts to absorb D.O.s into its ranks.

The growth in the osteopathic profession is apparent in the growing numbers of practitioners, particularly after the establishment of new osteopathic colleges in the 1970s. The number of practicing D.O.s in the United States increased from 8,410 in 1932 to 13,708 in 1960; it then fell slightly to 13,454 in 1970, largely because of the absorption of most California D.O.s into biomedicine. The number rose again to 18,820 in 1980, to 25,429 in 1986, and to 40,344 in 1997 (information obtained from the American Osteopathic Association).

THE DILEMMAS OF FUNCTIONING AS A
PARALLEL MEDICAL SYSTEM

Even though osteopathic medicine has improved its sociopolitical status and gained legitimacy as a parallel medical system to biomedicine, it continues to find itself in a precarious situation. Leaders of the osteopathic profession have successfully prevented the wholesale organizational absorption of their profession by biomedicine, and the profession has undergone tremendous growth since the 1970s, but it is uncertain whether or not these gains will be translated into a rejuvenation and a refinement of the osteopathic concept — the birthright of osteopathy, so to speak. Based upon a survey of D.O.s in a midwestern metropolitan area, Eckberg (1987) concluded that osteopathic physicians continued to exhibit the identity dilemma that New (1958, 1960) had detected nearly three decades earlier.

After the AMA opened up internships and residencies in biomedical hospitals to D.O.s in December 1968, a truce of sorts developed between the two professions. Today very few biomedical physicians function within osteopathic settings, but osteopathic physicians frequently practice in biomedical ones. Osteopathic hospitals, which tend to be smaller than their biomedical counterparts, are having difficulty filling their residencies because they are forced to offer residents salaries lower than those at biomedical hospitals (Ginzberg 1992). Young D.O.s face pressures to view themselves as less and less different from M.D.s. Eventual merger with organized biomedicine along the lines of what happened in California in 1961 still remains a possibility. Gevitz notes, "at the present time the number of D.O.'s who are actively in favor of a merger with the AMA appears to be comparatively small; however, there are a greater number who, while wishing to keep the profession autonomous, are in favor of their schools changing the degree awarded to an M.D. and wish to be allowed to list themselves in that manner" (1982: 146). The osteopathic profession has engaged in much soul-searching in recent decades as to whether or not it is a distinct entity from biomedicine at the philosophical and therapeutic levels. Wolinsky observes:

> Some osteopaths argue that they are modern-day physicians and that their training is no different than that of allopathic physicians. Others argue that osteopathy is quite different. They, however, often have difficulty identifying what is really different. (1988:250–51)

Many patients also have trouble distinguishing between the two types of medicine. In a survey of a rural community in central Michigan, Riley (1980) found that a substantial majority of his subjects did not perceive any difference between D.O.s and M.D.s in terms of practice, although they tended to regard biomedicine more favorably than osteopathic medicine.

Regardless of the views of individual D.O.s and their patients, the AOA has engaged in extensive public relations efforts to underscore that osteopathic physicians are authentic physicians and that osteopathic medicine constitutes a comprehensive and holistic form of health care. The osteopathic profession has been urging greater emphasis on OMT as a treatment and has increased research on its efficacy (Sprovieri 1993, 1995).

As a parallel system to biomedicine, however, osteopathic medicine faces immense structural uncertainties. Many biomedical schools have been making efforts to produce more primary-care physicians, and, ironically, the osteopathic profession has been undergoing an increasing trend toward specialization (Eckberg 1987). As Gevitz astutely observes, osteopathic medicine constitutes "potentially the most unstable [alternative medical system] in that, sociologically speaking, it is far more difficult for a 'parallel profession' to maintain its equilibrium when the profession it parallels no longer regards it as the enemy, when its members increasingly interact with the members of the other profession on terms of mutual respect, and when the differences between the two groups are no longer thought of by their members as highly significant" (1988b:155–56).

Ultimately, the future of both osteopathic medicine and biomedicine in the United States depends upon changes in the larger political economy of health care. The fact that osteopathic medicine has become an integral part of the increasing corporatization of medicine may mean that its subsequent development is in large part beyond the control of its practitioners.

4

Chiropractic as the Foremost Professionalized Heterodox Medical System

Chiropractic was the last of the heterodox medical systems that arose in the nineteenth century in response to popular protests against the perceived shortcomings of regular medicine. Unlike many of the other systems, such as homeopathy, botanic medicine or eclecticism, and osteopathy, which either disappeared, were absorbed by biomedicine, or adopted many of its premises and practices, chiropractic continues to function on the fringes of mainstream medicine. It constitutes the most visible and successful example of alternative medicine in the United States today, despite the fact that its history has been marked by considerable factionalism. Chiropractic may owe its success to the fact that, like biomedicine, it internalizes the American "value system of self-reliance, rugged individualism, pragmatism, atomism, privatism, emotional minimalism, and a mechanistic conception of the body and its 'repair'" (Stein 1990:20).

THE PHILOSOPHICAL PREMISES, DEVELOPMENT, AND SOCIAL ORGANIZATION OF CHIROPRACTIC

In contrasting their philosophy to the reductionist one of biomedicine, chiropractors often assert that they practice a form of health care which focuses on the treatment of the whole person. In reality, however, the holism of chiropractic is limited in that it relies heavily, like biomedicine and osteopathy, on notions such as the machine analogy. In all three systems,

> the body is viewed as a machine, in some cases a godgiven perfect machine, in other cases a chemical-physical machine. In both cases the body is seen as normally running without trouble: occasionally, however, it needs repair or adjustment. Chiropractic and osteopathic concern themselves with the structure and function of the machine. Healing occurs by making structural corrections. . . . Allopathic doctrines concern themselves with how the machine has been damaged by foreign parts, either injury, tumors, germs, or other invaders. Healing

67

takes place through the active intervention of alternative chemicals which purge the foreign parts and restore correct chemical balance. (McQueen 1978:74)

Furthermore, biomedicine, osteopathy, and chiropractic, at least in their original forms, are based on the idea that healing involves the removal of a single cause: a pathogen in the case of biomedicine, a lesion in the case of osteopathy, and a subluxation in the case of chiropractic. McQueen maintains that "the priority of the belief in a single cause has resulted in the downplaying of social factors in the etiology of disease" (1978:74). All three paradigms are compatible with capitalist ideology because they depoliticize the sources of disease. Willis suggests that chiropractic actually may be more congruent with capitalist ideology (at least industrial capitalist) than is biomedicine because it espouses more of an "engineering approach to health" in which "individuals are like machines which can be tinkered with to get back into good running order" (Willis 1983:198). Given that back injuries constitute a major source of productivity loss in capitalist societies, chiropractic care seeks to return the body to "good running order"—a requirement for producing profit (Willis 1983:198). Unlike biomedicine, however, it has not contributed to the growth of the medical-industrial complex, which includes pharmaceutical companies and high-technology medical equipment companies. By and large, chiropractic constitutes a low-technology approach to health care.

At the therapeutic level, the development of American chiropractic was shaped by the internecine battles between "straights"—those who wished to focus on spinal adjustment—and "mixers"—those who wished to incorporate other modalities from what is loosely termed naturopathy (e.g., physiotherapy, hydropathy, electrotherapy, colonic irrigation, dietetics, exercise, and vitamin therapy). Because of its extreme eclecticism, naturopathy provided chiropractic mixers with a ready source from which to add a wide variety of techniques to their treatment regimen.

Historian J. Stuart Moore (1993) has categorized chiropractors on the basis of therapeutic philosophy rather than on the scope of their practice and argues that the development of American chiropractic was marked by a fundamental division between the "harmonialists" and the "mechanical rationalists." The harmonialists, starting with D. D. Palmer himself, believed that Matter and Spirit are intricately intertwined. Like Andrew Taylor Still, the founder of osteopathy, Palmer drew upon tenets of magnetic healing, Spiritualism, and bonesetting in formulating his manual medical system. The harmonial chiropractors quickly assumed two "clearly distinguishable temperaments" (Moore 1993:99). Among the first group,

chiropractic became a substitute religion, supplying a comprehensive examination of reality, complete in itself with claims of divine powers, suffering saints and martyrs, and sacred writings and utterances from the prophets (the Palm-

68

ers) who provided the ultimate source of authority—all wrapped in a millennial eschatology. (Moore 1993:99)

Among the second group, which Moore suggests perhaps characterized the majority of harmonialists, chiropractic became transformed into a Christian approach to health.

The mechanical rationalists, by contrast, pursued scientific validation "by culling from chiropractic a more rational approach, appropriating the values of the mechanical medical marketplace of the early twentieth century" (Moore 1993:49–50). Some of these chiropractors viewed licensing as a means for attaining legitimacy, whereas others believed that such laws would limit the scope of their practice. One group of mechanical rationalists organized themselves into the National Association for Chiropractic Medicine, a body that requires its some 300 members to openly renounce the concept of sub-luxation and to restrict their practice to musculoskeletal ailments (Butler 1992:70).

In their efforts to achieve legitimacy and improved social status in the United States, chiropractors have adopted a wide variety of strategies, including establishing professional associations, colleges, patient support groups, and practice-building seminars, and conducting lobbying campaigns (Baer 1996). At the organizational level, the history of American chiropractic has seen the emergence of rival associations at both state and national levels.

In 1905, Solon M. Langsworthy organized the short-lived American Chiropractic Association as the first national chiropractic association. In response, B. J. Palmer established the Universal Chiropractors Association (UCA) a year later. The UCA conducted a concerted campaign to defend straight chiropractors arrested for practicing medicine without a license (Wardwell 1992: 98). B. J. became annoyed when the UCA began admitting mixers in 1913. He broke with the organization in 1926 and organized the Chiropractic Health Bureau, renamed the International Chiropractors Association (ICA) in 1941, which became known as the primary national organization of straight chiropractors. A group of mixers organized a new American Chiropractic Association (ACA) sometime in the early 1920s (Wardwell 1992:100). It merged in 1930 with scattered remnants of the UCA to form the National Chiropractic Association (NCA) and "soon became the largest chiropractor association as it moved to improve education, defend arrested chiropractors, and promote chiropractic through better licensing laws and public relations" (Wardwell 1992:100). After B. J.'s death in 1963, ICA Vice President Alan A. Adams left the organization and attempted to create yet another incarnation of the American Chiropractic Association. The newly constituted ACA incorporated the membership of the NCA, which dissolved, but attracted only about half of the ICA members. Subsequently, the ACA became associated with

69

mixers and the ICA with straights, though the distinction between the two types is no longer clear, if it ever was.

Since the late 1960s, a variety of external factors, related to chiropractic's drive for legitimacy, have moved the ICA and the ACA closer together. Leaders of the two associations decided that they needed to join forces to obtain recognition from various federal agencies and jointly prepared a white paper following the 1967 surgeon general's study on the possible inclusion of chiropractic care under Medicare (Wardwell 1980:36). After the federal government recognized the Council on Chiropractic Education (CCE), which was originally established by the ACA, as the official accrediting agency for chiropractic schools, the ICA accepted the authority of the council as well. In September 1983, over 250 chiropractors attended the first ACA-ICA National Legislative Conference in Washington, D.C. (American Chiropractic Association 1983). Until 1980 both the ICA and the ACA were headquartered in Des Moines, Iowa, but both organizations relocated to Washington, D.C., in keeping with the chiropractic profession's aim to obtain greater legitimacy and government support.

Some chiropractors believed that the ICA had departed from the principles of straight chiropractic and formed their own association and colleges. In 1976 Thomas Gelardi, who had founded the Sherman College of Chiropractic in Spartanburg, South Carolina, in 1973, formed the Federation of Straight Chiropractic Organizations (FSCO)—a third national faction composed of chiropractors whom their opponents refer to as "superstraights." It advocates "P, S, and U" (pure, straight, and unadulterated) chiropractic, purportedly taught and practiced as B. J. originally formulated it.

Many of chiropractic's internal conflicts have played themselves out in the formation of rival colleges. Wiese and Ferguson (1985) identified 392 different chiropractic colleges that have existed during the turbulent history of chiropractic education. According to Wardwell,

> When those for which there is no evidence of more than a year of operation are eliminated, the number is reduced to 188. Most of them probably produced few graduates. . . . The number of schools increased rapidly to their largest total between 1910 and 1926, and then contracted, particularly during the depression of the 1930s and World War II. Although veterans' educational benefits after World War II attracted more students, the number of schools continued to decline through 1970, largely through mergers, as the costs of the improved curricula exceeded the tuition that fewer students could bring in. (1992:91)

In the mid-1930s, John J. Nugent vigorously attacked those chiropractic schools that he regarded to be inferior and spearheaded an educational reform of chiropractic colleges that resulted in his appointment as the NCA's first director of education (Moore 1993:113–15).

In keeping with its sectarian and pecuniary tendencies, American chiropractic has drawn heavily upon both Protestant Evangelicalism and American entrepreneurialism. Chiropractors who were arrested and jailed for practicing medicine without a license during the first three decades of the twentieth century were viewed by their fellow practitioners as martyrs and saints. In the early 1920s, hundreds of chiropractors sang "Onward Christian Soldiers" in California on their way to jail (Gibbons 1977:143). The International Chiropractic Association endorsed the distribution of a "Chiropractic Prayer" that appeals to a higher power—an *Innate Intelligence, Life Force,* or *Dynamic Essentials*—for "help in the effective use of hands in order to ameliorate the pain in this troubled world" (Cowie and Roebuck 1975:59).

Whereas biomedicine has become an integral part of American corporate culture, chiropractic retains its initial commitment to the notion that the "common man" can rise from "rags to riches" by means of hard work and rugged, individualistic entrepreneurialism. In contrast to D. D. Palmer, who was a "dreamer," B. J. was an enterprising businessman, "a consummate salesman and showman" (Wardwell 1992:65), who solved the financial problems of the chiropractic school founded by his father. In addition to attracting thousands of students to the "Fountainhead" (the Palmer School), B. J. produced advertising brochures describing the "wonders" of chiropractic. He added business and advertising courses to the curriculum of the Palmer School of Chiropractic around 1920. B. J. and his faculty also wrote books and brochures and lectured widely on sales techniques and advertising. In a book titled *Questions and Answers about Chiropractic* (1952), B. J. wrote: "Q. What are the principal functions of the spine? A. 1) To support the head; 2) To support the ribs; 3) To support the chiropractor" (quoted in Weil 1983:130).

As a professionalized heterodox medical system, chiropractic has held out the promise of the American Dream for thousands of lower-middle-class and working-class individuals who, because of structural barriers, were denied access to careers in biomedicine. Although most of these were white males, a relatively high percentage of women chose to pursue a career in chiropractic in the early years of the profession. Three of the first 15 graduates of the Palmer Infirmary and Chiropractic Institute were women. In Washington, D.C., 5 of the 10 chiropractors listed in the 1913 and 1914 city directories were women. In 1919, the ratio was 16 of 33; in 1921, it fell slightly to 30 of 92. Although a proportion of one-third women was more typical nationwide, some areas remained higher; in 1925, 40 percent of the chiropractors in Kansas were women (Moore 1993:105).

Even more so than osteopathic students, chiropractic students came from relatively humble social origins. The Stanford Research Institute (1960) reported that most California chiropractors came from "families of modest means," and that 65 percent of them worked 20 hours or more per week while attending chiropractic school (comparable figures for osteopathic and bio-medical students were 17 percent and 1 percent, respectively). Fewer than 10 percent of the chiropractors had earned a bachelor's degree. In his study of students at New York's Columbia Institute of Chiropractic (CIC), Stern-berg found that most of them came from working-class families, and that the "American Dream value patterns seem[ed] very dominant in CIC's subcul-tural definition of the practice of chiropractic" (1969:268). Whereas the me-dian annual income at the time for chiropractors who had been practicing for 10 to 15 years was $28,400, the students anticipated earning a median income of $52,000. Based upon a questionnaire completed by 30 chiroprac-tors in three Ohio counties, White and Skipper reported that their respon-dents typically "were white, Protestant, male, and from lower-class origins in the midwestern section of the country" and enjoyed "a more comfort-able existence than that to which the chiropractors were accustomed while growing up" (1971:304). In contrast to the Waspish composition of the Ohio sample, Sternberg found that the CIC students were "not ethnically nor reli-giously typical of chiropractic" but were "much more heavily Jewish or Ital-ian" (1969:52). Research needs to be conducted on the matter of how Jews and Catholics fit into a profession with such strong Evangelical Protestant inclinations.

A 1978 study of 149 students at a Southern California chiropractic school presented the following social profile:

> The typical student is male, although 25 percent are female. He is between the ages of twenty-eight and thirty, although ages range from eighteen to fifty-six, single (47 percent) or married but with only one or two children. . . . Women are becoming increasingly attracted to the chiropractic arts, in part as a result of the recruiting of women by the profession and the schools, but more commonly younger women attend chiropractic school . . . .
>
> In obvious contrast to medical students, chiropractic students are from pri-marily working- and middle-class backgrounds: 40 percent of the fathers were skilled laborers, 15 percent small business owners, 14 percent managers or ex-ecutives, 19 percent professionals (which included chiropractors, medical doc-tors, teachers, engineers), 9 percent salesmen or clerical workers and 4 percent farmers. (Wild 1978:35–36)

Later studies suggested that people from somewhat higher socioeconomic brackets were beginning to be recruited into chiropractic. In a survey of 67 chiropractors in Nebraska, Rosenthal reported that 35.9 percent of his respondents "claim to have come from homes where the father was a pro-fessional or manager and 27% had fathers with some college experience" (1986:44). Another study of chiropractic students in the 1980s showed that they were younger than their counterparts in the past and that they had chosen chiropractic as an alternative to biomedicine or osteopathic medicine (McNamese et al. 1990). Recently, many chiropractic students have come from the related fields of physical education, nutrition, and nursing. Although there is an appreciable representation of "white ethnic" chiropractors in certain regions of the country, African Americans and other minorities are underrepresented. The Council on Chiropractic Education reported that of the 8,252 students enrolled in American chiropractic colleges in fall 1991, only 137, or 1.6 percent, were black (Wiese 1994:19).

Historically, chiropractic has recruited a fair number of its practitioners from the ranks of satisfied patients. According to Moore, "deliverance from a pain-wracked life, dramatic and compelling, often prompted a profound conversion to a way of health that not only sent converts into the streets proclaiming the glad news, but also convinced many to abandon their current livelihood and take up a chiropractic career as a means of testifying and ministering more directly to their newfound Way of Health" (1993:94).

THE NICHE OF CHIROPRACTIC WITHIN THE AMERICAN DOMINATIVE MEDICAL SYSTEM

When one considers the broad range of modalities utilized by the mixers and the fact that the membership of the ACA outnumbers that of the ICA by about three to one, it may appear on the surface that American chiropractic is evolving into a parallel medical system, traveling a pathway pioneered by osteopaths. Although the majority of mixers regard spinal adjustment as their primary therapeutic technique, as early as the 1930s many chiropractors were reportedly "as close to the medical camp as the osteopaths," and some even identified themselves as "chiropractic physicians" (Turner 1931: 205). By the 1920s, "progressives," such as those belonging to the Progressive Chiropractic Association of California, urged the inclusion of minor surgery, optometry, obstetrics, and general hospital work into the curricula of chiropractic schools (Turner 1931:142–46). Certain biomedical physicians played an influential role within American chiropractic. A. B. Herder, a biomedical physician, served as the first dean of faculty at the Palmer School of Chiropractic, and A. F. Walters, a Philadelphia surgeon and faculty member at the Medical College of the University of Pennsylvania, became a chiropractor who wrote and lectured extensively on his new profession (Schafer 1977: 26). Shortly after the turn of the twentieth century, the administration of the National School of Chiropractic, which evolved into the premier school of "mixer" chiropractic, "passed into the hands of a group of physicians, who became officers of the institution and occupied the majority of positions listed as professorships" (Gibbons 1981:237).

73

Despite the presence of biomedical physicians in both osteopathy and chiropractic, the osteopathic M.D.s appear to have had a different orientation from the chiropractic M.D.s. Whereas the former viewed themselves as reformers who wished to improve the dominant paradigm, the latter tended to be radical dissidents who felt that they had discovered a higher form of medical truth. According to Gibbons, "chiropractic journals are filled with evangelical accounts of M.D.s who took up their new calling" (1981:236). While a few M.D.s who converted to chiropractic possessed impeccable medical credentials, most had obtained degrees from the proprietary schools that existed in great number in the pre-Flexnerian era. Based upon their visit to the National School of Chiropractic in 1927, representatives of the AMA Council on Medical Education and Hospitals declared that the four physicians on the faculty lacked "any standing in the organized medical profession of America" (quoted in Gibbons 1981:240). Much the same could be said of A. T. Still and some of the regular physicians who followed him; nevertheless, the founder of osteopathy never castigated regular medicine with the same vengeance as did D. D. Palmer and his son, B. J. Aside from a few flirtations between chiropractic and biomedicine, chiropractors "have always been outsiders to the medical profession" (Wardwell 1978:9), and they have tended to regard themselves in this manner. B. J. Palmer's assertion that chiropractic constitutes "the antithesis of medicine" had a significant influence on the fate of the chiropractic profession, according to Wardwell (1978:10).

A study by the Stanford Research Institute concluded that in contrast to straights, who viewed themselves as drugless general practitioners, many mixers came to regard themselves as specialists not only in manipulative therapy but also in the treatment of a wide variety of other health problems. Consequently, they "have organized themselves into professional specialty societies with designations similar to those of medical and osteopathic specialists" (Stanford Research Institute 1960:30). Many chiropractors have expanded their practice beyond the bounds of manipulative therapy. A study conducted in the 1950s indicated that although musculoskeletal conditions constituted 46.8 percent of the conditions attended by chiropractors in comparison to 16.0 percent of those attended by osteopathic physicians and 13.6 percent of those attended by regular physicians, the chiropractors were also treating a wide variety of other complications, including hemorrhoids, cardiovascular conditions, varicose veins, congenital malformations, deafness, migraines, and headaches (Stanford Research Institute 1960:42). Pioneer chiropractors viewed obstetrics as a "natural extension of an alternative healing practice based upon physical therapeutics" (Gibbons 1982:27). Beginning in the early 1920s, spinal adjustment was used to treat the mentally disturbed in chiropractic sanatoriums and hospitals (Quigley 1983). Roth maintains that many chiropractic mixers "want to capture as much of the health therapy market as

74

they possibly can. . . . they have a series of brochures on a great many diseases to try to change the public stereotype that they are solely spinal manipulators and to sell the notion that they can treat a wide variety of illnesses and impairments" (1976:74).

At the same time, many chiropractors, particularly mixers, have come to view themselves as specialists within the American dominative medical system. Wardwell contends that, for both straights and mixers, "the vast majority of chiropractic treatment is more neuromuscular-skeletal conditions with perhaps 10 to 15 percent for organic conditions" (1982:217). Whereas mixers have been more likely to see their scope of practice as limited, straights have tended to view themselves as broad-spectrum practitioners (Wardwell 1980:36). It appears that while mixers prefer to view themselves as broad-spectrum practitioners, philosophically they have been more willing to come to terms with the fact that they function primarily as musculoskeletal specialists. Based upon questionnaires administered to 44 chiropractors in the Los Angeles metropolitan area, Coulter, Hays, and Danielson concluded that

> the most frequent recommendations are those most directly relevant to the complaints of back-related problems rather than general health and preventive care. These results seems to reflect the reality that practitioners are likely to recommend what is most relevant to what they are treating. The results suggest that extensive primary care is not being delivered by the sample of chiropractors (if primary care is meant as general and preventive health care and health promotion). (1996:108)

Overall, chiropractors have come to occupy a considerably more specialized niche within the American dominative medical system than have osteopathic physicians. This trend is apparent in the chiropractic hospitals and sanatoriums—such as the D. D. Palmer Memorial Hospital in Oklahoma City, Wisconsin General Chiropractic, and the Bakkum Chiropractic Hospital in Iowa—that existed between 1920 and 1960 (Gibbons 1980:16). These hospitals were considerably more limited in their scope of practice than were biomedical and osteopathic hospitals. The most famous chiropractic hospital was opened by Leo Spear in Denver during World War II. The demise of chiropractic hospitals—largely a consequence of the tremendous cost of constructing and operating hospitals without government funding and payments from third-party payers—effectively prevented chiropractors from functioning as comprehensive health care providers. Because chiropractic students are denied hospital training, chiropractors have functioned as "medical untouchables" with whom, until relatively recently, biomedical physicians refused to interact (Anderson 1981).

Evidence suggests that in rural areas, some chiropractors, if not many, function as drugless general practitioners (Stanford Research Institute 1960). One study showed that 40.7 percent of chiropractors practiced in communities with a population of under 25,000 (Foundation for the Advancement of Chiropractic Tenets and Science 1980:11). In some areas, they play the dominant "physician" role in the community (Krause 1977:44–45). Although chiropractors more often practice in rural and lower-income areas than do biomedical physicians, there are exceptions: in South Dakota, rural communities have fewer chiropractors than do urban areas (Kassak 1994).

Two contrasting orientations have developed in American chiropractic. In keeping with early chiropractic thought, the first regards chiropractic as a comprehensive or nearly comprehensive medical system, which includes general practice and specialty areas, including orthopedics, obstetrics and gynecology, proctology, and psychiatry. The second view, perhaps one reluctantly accepted by an increasing number of chiropractors, considers chiropractic as a limited or specialized practice which in time will gain full legitimacy, much in the same way that dentistry, optometry, and podiatry have.

THE ETHNOGRAPHIC STUDY OF CHIROPRACTIC

Several researchers have conducted ethnographic studies of chiropractic in either educational or clinical settings. In his observations at the Columbia Institute of Chiropractic (CIC) in New York City, Sternberg (1969) found that the majority of faculty and students repeatedly complained that the public and most of their patients perceived them as "back doctors." He reported that very few students used the college library and that the majority of students and faculty viewed basic science courses as "garbage courses." Aside from the clinic director, all of the other 20 faculty members taught part-time. In contrast to biomedical students, CIC students tended to be atomistic and generally did not interact after classes. In large part, this was due to the fact that the financial status of many students forced them to take full-time or part-time jobs that were unrelated to chiropractic. Sternberg maintained that CIC students quickly internalized the message that chiropractic was a besieged profession. On the whole, Sternberg's findings confirm the observation that chiropractic historically has functioned as a vehicle of upward social mobility for lower-middle-class and working-class people.

Cowie and Roebuck (1975) also documented the marginal status of chiropractors in an ethnographic study of a chiropractic clinic in a small southern town. In the course of his doctoral studies at Mississippi State University, Cowie obtained employment as a part-time chiropractic assistant in the clinic. The chiropractor's wife served as a full-time chiropractic assistant. The chiropractor and chiropractic assistant devoted much energy to "impression management," especially in the case of new patients, who often felt nervous

76

about seeking out a medical system that had so often been castigated by both biomedicine and the mass media. They attempted to create an ambience that combined professionalism and folksiness in both their demeanors and the furnishings of the waiting room. Pictures, signs, posters, and literature in the waiting room communicated the chiropractic message: the importance of maintaining one's body in good running order through a regular program of spinal adjustments. As Cowie and Roebuck observe,

> The practitioner was well aware of the situational difficulties faced by the new patient. Much of the backstage conversation between practitioner and staff involved discussions of the importance of the assistant-patient relationship. We were urged to "get involved with the patient." The general office duties of the assistant were incidental to the primary task of interaction stimulation. (1975:72)

When the new patient entered the adjustment area, the chiropractor assumed a friendly, easy-going stance in eliciting an understanding of the patient's ailment. He made a concerted effort to dispel common misunderstandings about chiropractic care. Stock explanations included the "vested interests of powerful medical lobbyists and an erroneous faith in the germ theory of disease" (Cowie and Roebuck 1975:83). At the beginning of the physical examination, the chiropractor told the patient to remain quiet so that they both could concentrate on the spine. He used X rays for three basic reasons: "(1) they provided a source of immediate and substantial income; (2) once the patient had spent that sum of money he [or she] usually committed himself [or herself] to at least a short series of appointments; and (3) the X rays offered much support to the statements made by the chiropractor concerning the patient's physical condition" (Cowie and Roebuck 1975:87). He categorized patients as falling into three types: "the one-timer or the one-shot patient," the problem patient, and the regular patient (Cowie and Roebuck 1975:114–27).

Despite his assorted marketing strategies, the practitioner earned a modest income which he did not feel was congruent with his professional expertise. He frequently sought advice from Sid E. Williams, a prominent chiropractic leader who had established the Life Chiropractic College in Marietta, Georgia, in 1974 and conducted practice-building seminars. The two had been fellow students at the Palmer College of Chiropractic. Despite a steady barrage of negative messages about his profession, the chiropractor felt that he had the "natural and Eternal Truths of chiropractic" on his side (Cowie and Roebuck 1975:111).

John L. Coulehan (1985a, 1985b), a biomedical physician with a strong interest in medical social science, conducted observations and interviewed 10 chiropractors in Pittsburgh. He maintained that, although clinical trials suggest that chiropractic treatment generally provides only short-term relief for musculoskeletal problems, the "clinical art" exhibited in the chiropractor-patient relationship tends to contribute greatly to healing.

Anthropologist Kathryn S. Oths concluded, based upon her fieldwork in a chiropractic office, that chiropractors rely upon psychotherapeutic techniques in their interactions with patients:

> Chiropractic functions to treat both psyche and soma. . . . Clients of the chiropractor seek help for somatic complaints which are often disguising problems of a psychological nature. The chiropractor explicitly treats the patient's physical complaints with no overt mention of his attention to patients' problems of living, yet patients frequently report doing better with job, family, and friends after being under the chiropractor's care for some time. . . . Patients also complained quite frequently about unsatisfactory medical care they had received from physicians and hospitals. (1992:92)

Based upon her observations of Dr. A, Oths (1994:92–93) delineated the following stages in the chiropractic-patient encounter:

(1) The *intake* or initial interview generally lasts from 8 to 20 minutes. This includes inquiries into past accidents and lifestyle and a brief introduction to chiropractic philosophy.
(2) The *initial orthopedic examination* immediately follows the intake. This lasts 12 to 20 minutes and consists of a series of range of motion and neurological tests.
(3) The *consultation* occurs a day or two following the initial encounter. At this time the chiropractor discusses his findings, including X rays, with the patient and significant others present.
(4) The first *spinal manipulation* lasts for 2 to 10 minutes.
(5) Periodic *reexaminations* may follow, particularly if the patient's condition has stabilized.

The chiropractor frequently translates biomedical terminology into lay terms that the patient can better understand.

ORGANIZED BIOMEDICINE'S CAMPAIGN TO SUPPRESS CHIROPRACTIC

Perhaps in part because chiropractic elicited much popular appeal, American biomedicine directed the severest of its attacks against heterodox medical systems toward chiropractic. As Wardwell observes, "more than osteopaths, who were considered to be irregulars and sectarian by orthodox medicine, chiropractors have been totally rejected as incompetent quacks or as hopeless

78

cultists" (1978:9). Sociologist Saul F. Rosenthal (1986:71–86) characterized the AMA's assault against chiropractic as a "holy war." In the early years of chiropractic, the AMA devoted little official attention to the new heterodox upstart. However, local physicians often provoked law-enforcement agencies to prosecute chiropractors for practicing medicine without a license. In response to the growing legal recognition of chiropractic around World War I, organized biomedicine embarked upon a concerted campaign to suppress chiropractic.

After World War I, the AMA Department of Investigation concentrated most of its resources against chiropractic (Cooper 1985:20). Morris Fishbein, secretary of the AMA and editor of the *Journal of the American Medical Association,* conducted a campaign in both professional and popular publications against chiropractic from 1924 to 1949 (see Fishbein 1932). Articles opposing chiropractic regularly appeared in biomedical journals. This campaign subsided somewhat during the Depression and World War II—a period when many chiropractic schools were forced to close and many of their graduates failed to pass basic science examinations.

Following the emergence of the mixers as the dominant chiropractic faction after World War II, the AMA adopted a more virulent posture toward chiropractic. In 1963 a Committee on Quackery was established to supplement the activities of the Department of Investigation. The Committee expressed its goal as being the "containment . . . and ultimately the elimination of chiropractic" (Trever 1972:4). In the late 1960s the AMA also sponsored an anti-chiropractic campaign and funded Ralph Lee Smith to write *At Your Own Risk: The Case against Chiropractic* (Peterson and Wiese 1995:194).

The AMA collaborated covertly with physicians in the Department of Health, Education, and Welfare in the preparation of a purportedly objective study of the potential incorporation of chiropractic services under Medicare (Cohen 1968). It formally labeled chiropractic "an unscientific cult" and forbade its members from associating with or referring patients to chiropractors. Successfully preventing initial congressional support of chiropractic services under Medicare,

> the AMA worked with the National Associations of Blue Shield Plans regarding coverage of chiropractic care, even in those states that had passed so-called 'insurance equality' laws. The AMA worked with the Health Insurance Association—a trade association of some 400 private insurance companies—to adopt policy statements that encouraged member insurance companies to cover those health-care practitioners whose methods were based on 'scientifically established methods.' (Null 1986:20)

In 1977 the California Committee against Health Fraud emerged as a successor to the AMA Coordinating Committee Conference on Health Information (Carter 1993:43). This body, which became the National Council against Health Fraud in 1984, was a major critic of chiropractic.

Chiropractic achieved a victory against the assault of organized biomedicine in the Wilk decision, evidence that it has achieved partial legitimation—a topic discussed in the following section (Wardwell 1992:168–78; Moore 1993: 131–37). In October 1976 Chester A. Wilk and four fellow chiropractors filed a suit against the AMA, the American Hospital Association, the American Academy of Orthopaedic Surgeons, five other medical associations (including the American Osteopathic Association), and four individuals, for allegedly violating the Sherman Antitrust Act by conspiring to eliminate chiropractic through refusal to consult with chiropractors. Perhaps in anticipation of a ruling against it, the AMA Judicial Council in 1978 ruled that M.D.s could accept referrals from and make referrals to chiropractors. The Wilk case first went to trial in Chicago in December 1980. In August 1987 Federal District Judge Susan Getzendanner found the AMA and its codefendants guilty of violating the Sherman Act. The AMA appealed the decision, but in early 1990 the 7th U.S. Circuit Court of Appeals upheld Getzendanner's findings. Despite this ruling, a number of biomedical physicians belonging to the Health Care Anti-Fraud Association continued the attack on chiropractic (Lisa 1994: 214–18).

THE PARTIAL LEGITIMATION OF CHIROPRACTIC: ACHIEVEMENTS AND LIMITATIONS

Licensing laws played a crucial role in the development of American chiropractic. In order to protect themselves from prosecution against laws prohibiting the practice of medicine by anyone other than an M.D. and to gain some degree of legitimacy, most chiropractors favored licensure, which was initially opposed by organized biomedicine. Some chiropractors felt ambivalent about licensing, however, because they realized that it could be used as a mechanism for restricting their scope of practice. In 1913 Kansas became the first state to enact a chiropractic statute; by 1938 all but seven states had passed chiropractic licensing laws. The last states to license chiropractors were New York (1963), Massachusetts (1966), Mississippi (1973), and Louisiana (1974). Wardwell maintains that "where organized medicine could not prevent chiropractic licensure, it sought the narrowest possible definition of its scope and control of the licensing process through its medical board" (1982:223). As a way of broadening their scope of practice, many mixer chiropractors obtained licenses as naturopaths. For many years, many mixer colleges offered their students the N.D. (Doctor of Naturopathy) diploma in addition to the D.C. (Doctor of Chiropractic). Chiropractic licensing laws vary widely in terms of the scope of practice that they permit. Oregon permits chiropractors to practice obstetrics, perform minor surgery, and sign birth and death certificates, while Washington State allows only spinal adjustment. Understandably, chiropractors prefer their own licensing boards to those dominated by biomedical physicians.

Although legislation recognizing chiropractic has existed in all 50 states since 1974, the manner in which chiropractors are regulated varies considerably from state to state. Regulation of chiropractic occurs in the form of medical boards that are monopolized or dominated by biomedical physicians; basic science boards that examine biomedical, osteopathic, and chiropractic students in the basic sciences as well as in clinical areas; all-chiropractic boards; and drugless practitioner acts. Licensure has played and continues to play a double-edged role in the development of American chiropractic.

In preparing students to pass basic science examinations and to meet state licensing requirements, chiropractic schools modified their curricula with the result that they began to resemble those of the biomedical schools. Ironically, as the chiropractic schools structured their programs so that their graduates could pass basic science examinations, "support for basic science boards declined from 17 states in 1950 to six states in 1979" (Wardwell 1982:224). In 1969 the ACA and ICA officially stated that subluxation was not the sole cause of nearly all diseases, as D. D. Palmer had claimed. Describing the transformation of chiropractic, Coburn and Biggs note that "one could claim that chiropractic, insofar as its theory is concerned, is becoming 'medicalized' in the sense of accepting the 'scientific medicine' model" (1986:1043). In becoming more acceptable in official circles, however, chiropractic has become enmeshed in that process through which "professionals" or "experts" become separated from those they originally served. Rather than treating primarily working-class and farm people, chiropractors now cater to a broad clientele, including substantial numbers of affluent professionals who can afford an increasingly expensive form of health care and tend to be less tolerant of bodily aches and pains than the working class (Kelner, Hall, and Coulter 1980:134–35). Like osteopathic medicine, chiropractic is also emulating the trend toward specialization characteristic of biomedicine. At the same time that chiropractic has evolved into a neuromuscular-skeletal speciality, it has developed an array of subspecialties in orthopedics, radiology, nutrition, and sports medicine. If chiropractors continue to be admitted to practice in hospitals, as has occurred in several states, they may also be seduced by the glamour of capital-intensive, high-technology medicine. Advertisements for medical technology appearing in chiropractic journals suggest that this trend may already be under way.

Despite vigorous opposition from organized biomedicine, chiropractic has undergone considerable legitimation since the early 1970s. As osteopathic physicians filled the vacuum left by regular physicians in primary care, they in turn left the treatment of musculoskeletal complications almost totally in the hands of chiropractors. Chiropractors have relied primarily on lobbying to obtain legal rights and third-party payments. In addition to the legitimacy obtained through licensure, American chiropractic has obtained additional government support. The process by which chiropractic obtained support from government agencies and private parties has not been fully explored. The federal government provided its first subsidy for chiropractic by paying for the schooling of World War I veterans (Gibbons 1980:18). Since the 1970s, governmental support for chiropractic has included (1) coverage for chiropractic care under Workers' Compensation in all 50 states and the District of Columbia, (2) the allowance of sick leave based upon a statement from a chiropractor for federal civil service employees, (3) federal income tax deductions for chiropractic care, and (4) coverage for chiropractic in all or nearly all states under Medicaid and Medicare. The chiropractic profession, however, has to date received only two research grants from the National Institutes of Health. Nevertheless, chiropractic schools have come to place increased emphasis on research and now employ a fair number of researchers with Ph.D.s in the health sciences. Ian Coulter, a Ph.D. sociologist and past president of the Canadian Memorial Chiropractic College in Toronto, and Joseph Keating, a Ph.D. psychologist, both work at the Los Angeles Chiropractic College in Whittier, California (personal communication).

In 1974 the United States Office of Education authorized the ACA Council on Chiropractic Education to act as the official accrediting agency of chiropractic colleges. Whereas no new chiropractic colleges were started between 1941 and 1972, the remainder of the 1970s saw the establishment of six new schools—two in California and one each in South Carolina, Georgia, Pennsylvania, and Texas—to bring the total number of chiropractic colleges in the United States to 17. The University of Bridgeport College of Chiropractic (est. 1991) is the newest of the chiropractic schools and the only one in the United States affiliated with a university—one operated by the Unification Church headed by the Reverend Sun Myung Moon.

Of the variety of factors, including concerted campaigns by chiropractors and their patients, that have contributed to government support of chiropractic in the United States, perhaps the most significant one is related to the relative inexpensiveness of low-technology chiropractic care compared to high-technology biomedicine. Chiropractic has caught the eye of an increasing number of health policy makers and convinced them that it provides a less costly and often more efficacious form of treatment for musculoskeletal conditions than does biomedicine. Indeed, reimbursements for low-technology health care are part of a larger effort to reduce inflation in health costs:

With the U.S. economy facing severe problems of inflation and intermittent recession, both corporations (who purchase the bulk of health insurance for the employees) and the Federal Government (which funds services for the poor and aged) are calling into question the amount of money being spent on medical care services. . . . Thus, health care expenditures appear unequivocally as a major factor limiting capital accumulation and a corporate strategy to reduce inflation in health costs is currently evident. Replacement of costly, high-technology medicine with cheaper, non-technological therapies is a major redirection advocated by proliferating medical-care evaluation studies. Corporations have developed an interest in holistic health, as *Forbes* magazine notes, "because it emphasizes more money-saving prevention and patient responsibility." (Berliner and Salmon 1980:141)

A study mandated by the U.S. Congress indicated that the annual educational cost per student in chiropractic colleges was less than that in biomedical, osteopathic, dental, pharmacy, podiatry, or veterinary colleges (Foundation for the Advancement of Chiropractic Tenets and Science 1980:44). With regard to costs of chiropractic care compared to other forms, the evidence is more equivocal. Studies sponsored by the Department of Industrial Relations in California (Wolf 1979), the Department of Industry in Wisconsin (Duffy 1978), the Iowa Industrial Commission (Velie 1978), and the Workers' Compensation Board of Oregon (Bergemann and Cichoke 1980) all showed that chiropractic treatment of back disability was less expensive and more effective in returning patients to the workplace than was regular medical care. Later studies also indicated that chiropractic care constituted a relatively cost-effective form of treatment compared to biomedical approaches (Alabama State Chiropractic Association 1993). A study in West Virginia, however, concluded that "chiropractic care of back and neck injury was not less costly or more effective in terms of work days lost in comparison to medical care" (Greenwood 1983). Despite the generally favorable findings of these studies,

The 1990s were relatively less supportive of chiropractic than the 1980s. The three principal problems were the expansion of HMOs [health maintenance organizations] and PPOs [preferred physicians' organizations], cutbacks in coverage by third-party payers and increased competition from the medical community. In spite of these obstacles, chiropractic continued to expand throughout the decade. (Caplan 1991:344)

Furthermore, some unions have also pressured insurers to pay benefits for chiropractic services.

While early statistics on the number of chiropractors fluctuate widely, it appears nevertheless that chiropractic has undergone considerable growth, particularly in recent decades. The 1990 Official Directory of the Federation of Chiropractic Licensing Boards listed 44,904 "resident D.C.s" in the United States (cited in Wardwell 1992:232).

The drive for professionalization has provided chiropractic with semi-legitimacy within American society, and it may now be evolving into what Wardwell has termed a "limited profession." Wardwell defines limited professions as "autonomous health-related professions that restrict their practices to part of the human body and, compared with M.D.s, limit the range of procedures, instruments, or techniques they use in treatment" (1992:43–44). Other examples of limited professions include dentistry, podiatry, optometry, and psychology. Although chiropractors still lack the legitimacy of these groups, they have gained some legitimacy within the context of the American dominative medical system. Chiropractors have for the most part been relegated to serving as musculoskeletal specialists, despite the desire on the part of many of them to function as drugless comprehensive practitioners. It is largely for this reason that chiropractors continue to rely upon the practice-building seminars and workshops that emerged in the early 1950s as an important mechanism for learning how to attract patients, instill confidence in themselves and their patients, learn office management techniques, and ultimately bolster their incomes (Baer 1996).

Moore contends that chiropractic "has moved into position as the orthodox, nontraditional approach to health—a type of orthodox unorthodoxy" that occupies a niche between biomedicine (and, I would add, osteopathic medicine) and the popular holistic health movement (1993:138). Whereas many biomedical physicians and some osteopathic physicians now work within the "capitalist commodity (industrialized, high technology, hospital-oriented)" mode of health care, the vast majority of chiropractors work within the "petty commodity (fee-for-service solo practitioners)" mode of health care (Rodberg and Stevenson 1977:106). According to Willis, chiropractic continues to be characterized largely by an "individualist mode of production" rather than a capital-intensive one (1983:163). Nevertheless, like other health services, chiropractic care has evolved into a medical commodity and a profitable enterprise. Chiropractors have emulated, and continue to emulate, the entrepreneurial, pecuniary practices of the competitive sector of the American political economy.

5

Naturopathy and Acupuncture as Secondary Professionalized Heterodox Medical Systems

Although medical historians and social scientists have written a fair amount on professionalized heterodox medical systems such as homeopathy, eclecticism, hydropathy, osteopathy, and chiropractic in the United States, naturopathy and acupuncture have received only passing mention. Twaddle and Hessler noted that naturopaths "have not yet received the attention of sociological research" (1987:191). Perhaps a major reason that social scientists have neglected American naturopathy is the perception that it would not last. Half a century ago, Wardwell predicted that naturopathy "apparently will soon disappear as a distinct therapeutic field," while noting that it should have attracted popular support because of its emphasis on natural foods, natural living, and a healthy environment (1951:39). Roth referred to naturopathy as an example of a dying health movement attempting "a last ditch struggle to survive" (1976:121). The future of American naturopathy remains uncertain, but there are a number of indications that it has entered into a period of rejuvenation: the modest growth of four-year naturopathic colleges in Seattle and Portland, Oregon; the recent establishment of four-year naturopathic colleges in Arizona and Connecticut; the formation of the American Association of Naturopathic Physicians; and the licensure of naturopaths in several states.

Unlike American naturopathy, which emerged around the turn of the twentieth century, American acupuncture as a professionalized heterodox medical system is a much more recent phenomenon. Like the rejuvenation of naturopathy, the development of acupuncture has overlapped with the rise of the holistic health movement. Acupuncture has obtained the greatest level of public recognition and political legitimation in California, where about half of all the licensed acupuncturists in the United States presently practice. The drug abuse and AIDS epidemics have contributed to increased American interest in acupuncture following reports of its effectiveness in drug treatment.

THE EMERGENCE OF AMERICAN NATUROPATHY

In contrast to other professionalized medical systems, such as homeopathy, osteopathy, and chiropractic, naturopathy has never had a well-integrated philosophical core or a specific regimen of treatment. Nevertheless, some general beliefs underlie the system. Naturopaths regard disease as a response to bodily toxins and imbalances in a person's social, psychic, and spiritual environment; germs are not the cause of disease per se but rather are parasites that take advantage of the body when it is in a weakened state. Because they believe that the healing power of nature, the *vis mediatrix naturae*, can restore one to health, naturopaths emphasize preventive health, education, and client responsibility. Their specific therapeutic approaches, however, have varied historically and cross-culturally (Pizzorno 1996). In the past, many naturopaths relied heavily on water treatments, colonic irrigation, dietetics, fasting, and exercise. While some naturopaths continue to advocate these modalities, others draw upon acupuncture, spinal manipulation, homeopathy, herbalism, vitamin therapy, faith healing, and even Ayurvedic and Chinese medicine. According to Bloomfield, "naturopathy for some people means *all* the forms of non-allopathic medicine which depend on 'natural' remedies and treatments" (1983:116). In many ways, American naturopathy emerged as the heir of the nineteenth-century hygiene movement, which drew upon the ideas of popular health reformers like Sylvester Graham, John Kellogg, and various advocates of hydropathy and hygeiotherapy, as well as the healing techniques of Father Sebastian Kneipp (Nissenbaum 1980; Whorton 1982).

While some naturopaths trace their practice back to Hippocrates and the medical system of ancient Egypt, the more immediate root of twentieth-century naturopathy is the tradition of health spas, which were widespread in central Europe in the eighteenth and nineteenth centuries. American naturopathy appears to have derived most directly from the Kneipp water societies and spas established shortly before the turn of the century; these, in turn, grew from an earlier movement called hygeiotherapy, a refinement of hydropathy. According to Whorton, naturopathy "differed in no important way from a refinement of . . . hygeiotherapy" (1985:45). Russell Trall, a physician who rejected allopathy for hydropathy, described hygeiotherapy as a system that "adopts all the remedial appliances in existence, with the single exception of poisons" (quoted in Whorton 1985:41), including massage, electrotherapy, diet, exercise, fresh air, and cleanliness. Although hygeiotherapy had virtually disappeared by the time of Trall's death in 1877, it underwent a resurgence in the 1890s in the form of Kneippism.

The Kneipp water societies were established after the heyday of American hydropathy, which also drew upon the ideas of Vincenz Priessnitz, an

86

Austrian peasant who administered cold water applications to stimulate vital organs (Weiss and Kemble 1967; Legan 1987). Father Sebastian Kneipp, a renowned Bavarian hydropath, modified Priessnitz's methods (described in chapter 1), supplementing them with the use of herbs. Father Rouge introduced Kneippism into New Orleans in June 1893 at the Mt. Carmel Orphan Asylum (Weiss and Kemble 1967:101). Kneippism was also brought to the United States by Benedict Lust. When Lust (1872–1945), a German immigrant to the United States, became consumptive, he returned home and was cured by the Kneipp treatment. He became a disciple of Kneipp, from whom he received a commission to start a society, school, and magazine (Weiss and Kemble 1967:107). He established the Kneipp Water-Cure Institute in Brooklyn in 1895, formed the first Kneipp water-cure society in Jersey City, New Jersey, in 1896, and began editing the *Kneipp Water Cure Monthly* in 1900 (Cody 1985:9). Kneipp societies were established in Manhattan, Brooklyn, Boston, Chicago, Cleveland, Denver, Cincinnati, Philadelphia, Columbus, Buffalo, Rochester, New Haven, Mineola (Long Island), New Mexico, San Francisco, and many other places (Wendel 1951:157). Kneippism attracted an assortment of medical heretics, including homeopaths, herbalists, and lay practitioners.

Lust purchased the term "naturopathy" from the hydropath John Scheel, who coined the term in 1895 to describe his medical system (Pizzorno 1996: 165). As Andrew Taylor Still and D. D. Palmer did in the case of their medical systems, Lust identified divine inspiration as the ultimate source of his system. He asserted that "naturopathy comes from the heart of Nature through the heart of man to the heart of God" (quoted in Kirchfeld and Boyle 1994: 193). Lust established the American School of Naturopathy in New York City in 1901. Louisa Lust, Benedict's wife, served as an instructor at the college (Kirchfeld and Boyle 1994:224). Lust also formed the Naturopathic Society of America (NSA) on December 2, 1902, in New York City and disbanded the Kneipp societies. Despite the name change, "hydropathy remained an important element in naturopathic medicine in the early twentieth century" (Brown 1987:226). Lust had many associations with German American physicians and earned a D.O. degree in 1898 from the Universal Osteopathic College of New York, an N.D. (Doctor of Naturopathy) degree in 1904 from the Eclectic and Naturopathic College, and an M.D. degree in 1914 from the Eclectic Medical College of New York (Cody 1985:10; Miller 1985: 56). The NSA was renamed the American Naturopathic Association in 1919 and billed as an organization "comprised of Graduates from Nature Cure, Hydrotherapy, Diet, Chiropractic, Osteopathy, Mechanotherapy, Neuropathy, Electropathy, Mental and Suggestive Therapeutics, Phototherapy, Heliotherapy, Phytotherapy and other rational and progressive schools of Natural Healing" (quoted in Wendel 1951:38).

Weil maintains that naturopathy "emerged slowly and without clear definition from an informal grouping of people who shared certain beliefs about health and medicine.... In some ways, the original naturopaths were glorified hygienists, who felt that clean living was the way to good health—hence the emphasis on fresh air, good diet, water, light, herbs, and other simple measures" (1983:138). Other naturopaths also established schools during the first three decades of the twentieth century. The number of naturopathic schools during this period fluctuated and is difficult to determine exactly. Zeff maintains that "by the 1930s there were about two dozen schools, and by some accounts, as many as 40,000 practitioners" (1996:59). Carl Schultz, another German immigrant, organized the Association of Naturopathic Physicians of California in 1901 and established the Naturopathic Institute Sanitorium in 1904 and later the Naturopathic College of California (Kirchfeld and Boyle 1994:212). Henry Lindlahr, a native of Germany and graduate of the National Medical University, established a sanatorium in 1903 in Elmhurst, Illinois, and shortly thereafter a clinic and food store on State Street in Chicago and the Lindlahr College of Natural Therapeutics (Wendel 1951:138; Cody 1985: 16). In 1908 he began to publish *Nature Cure Magazine* and the five-volume *Philosophy of Natural Therapeutics.* Lindlahr appears to have been second only to Lust in terms of fame in American naturopathic circles (Kirchfeld and Boyle 1994:227–50).

A 1927 AMA study listed twelve naturopathic schools with a total of fewer than 200 students (Reed 1932:66–68). These included the First National University of Naturopathy in Newark, New Jersey; the Naturopathic College in Philadelphia; and the Blumer College of Naturopathy in Florida. Pennsylvania at one time had five naturopathic schools (*American Association of Naturopathic Physicians Quarterly Newsletter* 1[2] 1986). Most early naturopaths in the Pacific Northwest referred to their medical system as "sanipractic." The American University of Sanipractic was opened in Seattle in 1920, and the Universal Sanipractic College was opened there in 1922 (Whorton 1986). Sierra States University of Naturopathy was established in Los Angeles in 1927 (*Journal of Naturopathic Medicine*, June 1966).

During the heyday of American naturopathy, naturopaths were licensed to practice in 25 states (Finken 1986:41). Estimates of the number of naturopaths during the 1920s and 1930s vary considerably. Reed (1932:62) put the number of naturopaths and related practitioners in the United States during the early 1930s at about 2,500, but Whorton (1986:19) estimated that there were some 400 "sanipractors" in Washington State alone in 1925. Although the American Naturopathic Association served as the principal naturopathic association, naturopathy has been plagued throughout most of its existence by organizational rivalry, fragmentation, and lack of national leadership.

In his undeniably jaundiced overview of "healing cults" in America, Reed observed that "the relationship between naturopathy and chiropractic are most close" (1932:62). Whereas osteopaths, in their efforts to become broad-spectrum practitioners, incorporated many aspects of biomedicine, many chiropractors also tended to expand their range of healing modalities by borrowing primarily from naturopathy. According to Reed, American naturopathy attained importance "contemporaneously with the development of 'mixing' in chiropractic" (1932:63). Naturopathy provided chiropractic mixers with a wide variety of techniques to add to their treatment regimens, and many mixer schools offered their students N.D. as well as D.C. degrees. Furthermore, many naturopathic schools taught chiropractic techniques and granted D.C. degrees. The Central States College of Naturopathy (also known as the Central States College of Physiatrics) in Ohio granted a Doctor of Mechanotherapy, or the N.D. for registration in other states, before it closed down sometime between 1966 and 1968 (Homola 1963:76). Reed asserts that "many naturopaths are former chiropractors—chiropractors who began using so many other healing methods that they ceased to call themselves chiropractors" (1932:63).

THE DECLINE OF AMERICAN NATUROPATHY

Various scholars have attempted to explain the decline, beginning in the 1940s, of American naturopathy. Wardwell argues that it lacked a specific therapeutic focus comparable to chiropractic adjustment and a charismatic leader such as B. J. Palmer "around whom, or in opposition to whom, the field could mobilize" (1951:39). Another factor was the growing disconnection between chiropractic and naturopathy. In the early twentieth century, chiropractic "mixers," who combined spinal manipulation with a wide array of therapeutic modalities, had found in naturopathy a mechanism by which to legally circumvent restrictive chiropractic laws in many states. Wardwell described the situation in the first half of the century as follows:

> Much as chiropractic leaders would like to see the awarding of N.D. degrees by chiropractic schools abandoned, they are faced with the realistic situation that chiropractors sometimes engaged in a wider scope of practice and with greater immunity from legal interference by registering as naturopaths. Hence, there is pressure on chiropractic schools to continue to make the N.D. degree available to students intending to practice in such states. (1951:137)

As a growing number of states dropped naturopathic licensing and/or permitted chiropractors a wide scope of practice, the original rationale followed by chiropractic schools for granting N.D. degrees lost relevancy. Wardwell notes that "when mixer [chiropractic] schools gave up naturopathy in mid-century, their programs became less comprehensive and probably less compatible with traditional medicine than they had previously been" (1982:244). The Los Angeles College of Chiropractic dropped its N.D. degree around 1948 and the National Chiropractic College in Illinois around 1950 (Homola 1963:75–76). The Western States College of Chiropractic in Portland was the last of the chiropractic schools to drop the N.D. degree when it did so in 1957.

Cody argues that the advent of "miracle drugs," the impact of World War II on health care, and the death of Benedict Lust in 1945 all contributed to the decline of American naturopathy (1985:21). Lust's ANA splintered into six different organizations during the mid-1950s. The primary organizations among these were the American Association of Naturopathic Physicians (AANP), the successor to the ANA (which had changed its name in 1950 to the American Naturopathic Physician and Surgeon's Association), and the National Association of Naturopathic Physicians, the American branch of the International Society of Naturopathic Physicians, which had been established after Lust's death by M. T. Campanella of Florida (Cody 1985:22). According to Cody,

> By 1955, the AANP, as it ultimately became known, had recognized only two schools of naturopathic medicine, those being the Central States College of Physiatrics in Eaton, Ohio, under the leadership of H. Riley Spitler, and the Western States College of Chiropractic and Naturopathy located outside of Portland, Oregon, under the leadership of R. A. Budden. (1985:22)

From 1940 to 1963, the AMA engaged in a systematic attack upon alternative medical systems, particularly chiropractic but also naturopathy. Since many naturopaths practiced under chiropractic licenses, "the medical establishment treated naturopathy and chiropractic as the same . . . [and thereby] the tactics used against each stemmed from strategies developed by the AMA to eliminate both from the health-care system" (Lisa 1994:272). After World War II severe limitations were placed on naturopaths through court decisions. The Tennessee legislature declared the practice of naturopathy a gross misdemeanor (Miller 1985:57). In 1953 the attorney general of Texas ruled the licensure of naturopaths unconstitutional (*American Association of Naturopathic Physicians Quarterly Newsletter* 1[3] 1986:4). Spurred on by lobbying from organized biomedicine, the Georgia legislature eliminated the naturopathic board of examiners in 1956 (Lisa 1994:268). Florida, which had first licensed naturopaths in the 1920s, ended licensure for them in 1959. California passed a "sunset" law in 1964 which permitted previously licensed naturopaths to practice but prohibited the granting of new naturopathic licenses (*American Association of Naturopathic Physicians Quarterly Newsletter* 2[5] 1987:3). By 1958 only five states (Arizona, Colorado, Connecticut, Virginia, and Utah) provided separate licensure for naturopaths, although a few states licensed them under drugless healer laws (Homola 1963:75). Ultimately, the decline of naturopathy must be viewed as a result of the growing hegemonic influence of biomedicine and the absence of relatively strong national organizations and lobbying campaigns—both of which chiropractic had managed to develop.

Despite its weakened position by mid-century, naturopathy found a stronghold of sorts in the Pacific Northwest, a region that has repeatedly provided a sanctuary for maverick social movements and alternative medical systems. As Whorton aptly argues,

> The green, unspoiled environment and the public's health consciousness were an inspiration . . . to local natural healers and an attraction to outside ones. The boom in population and the economy exerted another type of magnetism. And finally, there was the legal environment, which featured a medical licensing policy so liberal as to practically invite every imaginable species of quack and cultist to migrate to the region. . . . competition from unorthodox practitioners had been a thorn in the side of the regular profession from its very start in the area. (1986: 15)

Whereas most other state governments either refused to grant legal recognition to naturopathy or dropped former licensing laws permitting it, Washington and Oregon continued to provide a relatively open environment for sanipractors or naturopaths.

In response to the plans of the Western States College of Chiropractic to drop its N.D. program, Charles Stone, Frank Spaulding, and W. Martin Bleything established the National College of Naturopathic Medicine (NCNM) in Portland, Oregon, in 1956 (National College of Naturopathic Medicine 1987–1989:12). NCNM opened a campus in Seattle in 1959, and in 1973 established a collaborative program with the College of Emporia in Kansas, which provided NCNM students with two years of basic science courses. Kansas Newman College took over the program for several years before it reverted back to the NCNM campuses in Portland and Seattle. Although various naturopathic "degree mills" operated here and there during the early 1970s, the NCNM remained the sole four-year naturopathic school during that period. It suffered from financial problems, however, and in 1976 the NCNM campus in Seattle closed its doors.

THE REJUVENATION OF NATUROPATHY IN THE CONTEXT OF THE HOLISTIC HEALTH MOVEMENT

While it appeared that American naturopathy was indeed at a low ebb in the early 1970s, signs of a reversal in the tide appeared by the end of the decade. Naturopathy was in a sense preadapted for the holistic health movement that emerged in the early 1970s—a movement that emphasizes holism and a wide array of natural therapeutic approaches. In 1978 three NCNM graduates and an administrator established the John Bastyr College of Naturopathic Medicine (JBCNM), now Bastyr University, in Seattle (Weeks 1985/1986). John Bastyr, the namesake of the new college, had established a naturopathic practice in Seattle during the Depression. Under the presidency of Joseph Pizzorno, JBCNM opened a clinic in the University District of Seattle in 1978, graduated its first class in 1982, and in 1983 received Candidacy for Accreditation by the Northwest Association of Schools and Colleges, which was investigating the possibility of accreditation—a first for the naturopathic profession.

In the fall of 1979, another four-year naturopathic school, the Pacific College of Naturopathic Medicine (PCNM), opened its doors in Monte Rio, California (Pacific College of Naturopathic Medicine catalog, n.d.). According to a JBCNM faculty member, PCNM was mismanaged; it closed shortly after moving its operations to San Rafael, California, in order to be closer to a densely populated area. The lack of naturopathic licensure in California, which forced naturopaths to practice under acupuncture licenses, undoubtedly also contributed to the demise of PCNM.

Several other naturopathic or natural therapeutic schools also opened up in the 1970s and in later years in the United States. These include the Arizona College of Naturopathic Medicine; the American College of Naturopathic Medicine in Oregon; the Natural Therapeutics College in Mesa, Arizona; Dr. Jay Sherer's Academy of Natural Healing in Santa Fe, New Mexico; the New Mexico School of Natural Therapeutics; and the North American College of Natural Sciences in Mill Valley, California. Most of these institutions require or required less than four years of training. The Hallmark Naturopathic College in Sulphur, Oklahoma, offers correspondence courses in naturopathy, herbology, reflexology, aromatherapy, Native Medicine, and biologic ionization technology through its Web site.

In 1993 the Southwest College of Naturopathic Medicine and Health Sciences opened in Scottsdale, Arizona, joining the JBCNM and the NCNM as the only four-year naturopathic colleges in the United States. The school now has its campus in Tempe and its clinic in Scottsdale and offers a certificate in acupuncture in addition to the N.D. A fourth four-year naturopathic college opened its doors in 1997 at the University of Bridgeport (Connecticut)—this private institution, which recently came under control of the Unification Church, also operates the only university-based chiropractic college in the United States. The Professors World Peace Group, a Unification Church front organization, infused $50 million into the institution in exchange for control of the board of trustees (Clarkson 1997:56–59). In 1995, the University of Bridgeport granted the Reverend Sun Myung Moon an honorary doctorate. Given that many younger naturopaths tend to be politically liberal, it will be interesting to see what type of relationship they will have with an ultraconservative religious sect with whom a segment of the naturopathic profession has formed an alliance. Apparently, ecclesiastical and heterodox medical politics sometimes creates strange bedfellows.

Graduates of the JBCNM and NCNM as well as other naturopaths formed the American Association of Naturopathic Physicians (AANP), which held its first annual convention in Scottsdale, Arizona, in fall 1986 (*Holistic Medicine: Newsletter of the American Holistic Medical Association*, January/February 1988). Whereas only 30 people attended the first AANP convention, some 300 people, most of them JBCNM and NCNM students, attended the second AANP convention at the Alderbrook Inn on Hood Canal, an inlet of Puget Sound in Washington State (*American Association of Naturopathic Physicians Quarterly Newsletter* 3 [5] 1988). The AANP has 24 state associations (Alaska, Arizona, California, Colorado, Connecticut, Florida, Hawaii, Idaho, Maine, Massachusetts, Minnesota, Montana, Nebraska, New Hampshire, New Jersey, New Mexico, North Carolina, Oregon, Pennsylvania, South Dakota, Texas, Utah, Vermont, and Washington) and associations in the District of Columbia and Puerto Rico. It reportedly has about 750 members, and it publishes the *Journal of Naturopathic Medicine* (Collinge 1996:132). The AANP established the Council of Naturopathic Education, which received federal recognition in 1987. The council has granted accreditation to both Bastyr University and the National College of Naturopathic Medicine and candidacy for accreditation to the Southwest College of Naturopathic Medicine but has not yet recognized the University of Bridgeport College of Naturopathic Medicine. The Naturopathic Licensing Examination (NPLEX) developed by the council has received acceptance as a licensing examination in Arizona, Connecticut, Washington State, Washington, D.C., and British Columbia.

Naturopathic licensing laws now exist in 12 states (Alaska, Arizona, Connecticut, Florida, Hawaii, Maine, Montana, New Hampshire, Oregon, Utah, Vermont, and Washington). Naturopaths were "sunsetted" in California in 1964, but they often practice under an acupuncture or chiropractic license. Since most states do not register them, it is difficult to determine the number of practicing naturopaths. A "Naturopathic Doctor List" compiled by the AANP in the late 1980s indicated 1,044 naturopaths in the United States, with Oregon (215), Washington (210), California (120), Arizona (94), and Florida (77) topping the list. Zeff (1996) reported that there were some 1,500 licensed naturopathic physicians in the country in the mid-1990s.

AMERICAN ACUPUNCTURE AS AN EMERGING
PROFESSIONALIZED HETERODOX MEDICAL SYSTEM

Despite its Johnny-come-lately status, acupuncture has exhibited an even more marked pattern of growth than naturopathy. Acupuncture, which has been used for over 5,000 years as part of traditional Chinese medicine, gained broad popular attention in the United States following the lifting of the Bamboo Curtain in 1971, which opened relations between the governments of the People's Republic of China (PRC) and the United States. Two significant factors contributed to this attention (Wolpe 1985). The first was the treatment of *New York Times* columnist James Reston with acupuncture to alleviate the significant pain he experienced after undergoing an appendicitis operation while on tour in China. The second was the publication of glowing reports on the efficacy of acupuncture by a select group of American physicians who visited the PRC. Since then, the federal government has encouraged research on acupuncture, and scientific journals have published scores of articles on it. The first acupuncture clinic in the United States opened in New York City in July 1972, but it was shut down a week later—the practitioners were charged with practicing medicine without a license. Before it closed, the busy clinic had treated some 500 patients (Weiss and Lonnquist 1997:229).

Although some biomedical physicians, osteopathic physicians, chiropractors, and naturopaths now employ acupuncture, generally as an adjunct therapy, acupuncture is quickly evolving into a professionalized heterodox medical system in its own right in some areas of the country. In the mid-1990s an estimated 3,000 M.D.s and D.O.s in the United States employed acupuncture, but there were also several thousand nonbiomedical licensed acupuncturists in the country (Weiss and Lonnquist 1997:230).

LICENSING, CERTIFICATION, AND
REGISTRATION AND PUBLIC RECOGNITION OF
NONBIOMEDICAL ACUPUNCTURISTS

Beginning in the early 1970s, nonbiomedical acupuncturists, the majority of whom were Asian, began lobbying for laws that would legally recognize them in some capacity (Kao and McRae 1990:269). Organized biomedicine resisted their efforts by initiating a two-fold strategy: designing research to incorporate acupuncture into biomedicine as an adjunct therapy, and promoting legislation and propaganda to wrest acupuncture from nonbiomedical acupuncturists (Wolpe 1985:413–15). After forty states passed laws limiting acupuncture to M.D.s and D.O.s, nonbiomedical acupuncturists mounted a relatively successful counter-offensive. The American Association of Acupuncture and Oriental Medicine (AAOM) was established in 1981 and serves as an umbrella organization to coordinate legislative and research efforts. It reportedly has over 1,600 members (Collinge 1996:52). The National Commission for the Certification of Acupuncture (NCCA) represents about 2,000 nonbiomedical acupuncturists (Baer and Good 1998:51). Other organizations promoting acupuncture include the Council of Colleges of Acupuncture and Oriental Medicine (CCAOM)(est. 1982), the National Accreditation Commission for Schools and Colleges of Acupuncture and Oriental Medicine, and the National Acupuncture and Oriental Medicine Alliance. The Society for Acupuncture Research operates at a national level, and CCAOM promotes acupuncture research in California. While the AAOM still appears to constitute the main acupuncture organization in the United States, a bitter split within acupuncture several years ago led to the birth of the Alliance, which has more members in some states than does the AAOM (personal communication with Claire Cassidy). The split was prompted by the tendency on the part of acupuncture leaders in California to view acupuncture as an adjunct of biomedicine.

Nevada was the first state to establish a Board of Oriental Medicine (Chow 1984:134). This may be because in Nevada, neither biomedical physicians, physical therapists, nor chiropractors are qualified to practice acupuncture (Cargill 1994:152). By 1978 500 people, most of them nonbiomedical practitioners, had been licensed as acupuncturists in California (Wolpe 1985:419). In 1979 they were declared primary health care practitioners and are covered by Medi-Cal, California's Medicaid program. The State of California Acupuncture Committee administers licensing examinations for acupuncturists. A subcommittee of the Medical Board of California, it consists of 11 members, two of whom must be physicians and surgeons with at least two years of experience in acupuncture and four of whom are neither licensed acupuncturists nor physicians.

In addition to Nevada and California, other states that legally recognized nonbiomedical acupuncturists fairly early on were Florida, Hawaii, Montana, New Jersey, and New York (Chow 1984:133). By 1998, nonbiomedical acupuncturists had achieved licensure, certification, or registration in 34 states as well as the District of Columbia. Most of the East Coast and West Coast states license or certify nonbiomedical acupuncturists, whereas most of the interior states do not (Baer and Good 1998:51). The states legally recognizing nonbiomedical acupuncturists in some sort of capacity are Alaska, Arizona, Arkansas, California, Colorado, Connecticut, Florida, Hawaii, Illinois, Iowa, Louisiana, Maine, Maryland, Massachusetts, Montana, New Hampshire, Nevada, New Jersey, New Mexico, New York, North Carolina, Oregon, Pennsylvania, Rhode Island, South Carolina, Tennessee, Texas, Utah, Vermont, Virginia, Washington, West Virginia, and Wisconsin. In New Mexico, acupuncturists have legal recognition as Doctors of Oriental Medicine. The Office of Alternative Medicine (1992), which falls under the supervision of the director of the National Institutes of Health, reported the existence of some 6,500 licensed acupuncturists in this country, about half of whom were registered in California and some 1,600 of whom were members of the American Oriental Body Work Therapy Association.

Educational requirements for acupuncturists vary widely:

> Montana, for instance, requires a total of 105 hours in anatomy, biochemistry, microbiology or bacteriology, pharmacology, physiology, chemistry, and materia medica, but requires no training in traditional Chinese medicine. Nevada, on the other hand, requires three years of acupuncture training (1,400 hours or more) plus three years of practice, and requires that both physicians and nonphysicians pass an examination in acupuncture and traditional Chinese medicine. (Chow 1984:133)

Some states permit M.D.s and D.O.s to practice acupuncture without additional training. Other states require M.D.s and D.O.s to obtain some acupuncture training before practicing it. Some states permit, at least with additional training, physicians' assistants, dentists, podiatrists, chiropractors, and even naturopaths to practice acupuncture. Many states which have not passed licensing laws for nonbiomedical acupuncturists reportedly tolerate their sub-rosa practices. Arkansas and Tennessee do not even have rulings as to whether acupuncture falls within the definition of the practice of medicine. Wyoming does not regulate acupuncture at all.

Given that chiropractors, naturopaths, and other alternative practitioners have often, at least in the past, had difficulty obtaining compensation from insurance companies, passage of the California Insurance Law has been important for helping acupuncture to become a professionalized heterodox medical system. The law stipulates that insurance companies in California must provide policies that cover acupuncture treatment administered by either a physician or a licensed acupuncturist, but exempts health maintenance organizations (HMOs), preferred physicians' organizations (PPOs), and self-insured companies from this requirement. Nevertheless, Kaiser Permanente, the largest HMO in the United States, covers acupuncture but not chiropractic as a part of physical therapy (Kritz 1994:120). Despite a tendency by many alternative practitioners toward professionalization, others resist this process for a variety of reasons. Some acupuncturists ignore or circumvent licensing requirements in California and elsewhere. Practitioners of Chinese medicine often are located in Chinatowns and practice in back rooms of gift shops, where they treat low-income Chinese patients.

Table 3   Institutions Offering a Master's Degree in Acupuncture

Institution	Location
Acupuncture and Herbal Medicine College, Tai Hsuan Foundation	Honolulu, HI
American College of Traditional Chinese Medicine	San Francisco, CA
Bastyr University	Seattle, WA
Emperor's College of Traditional Chinese Medicine	Santa Monica, CA
Five Branches Institute: College of Traditional Medicine	Santa Cruz, CA
International Institute of Chinese Medicine	Santa Fe, NM
Keimyung Baylo University	Anaheim, CA
Kyung San University	Garden Grove, CA
Meiji College of Oriental Medicine	San Francisco, CA
Midwest Center for the Study of Oriental Medicine	Racine, WI
New England School of Acupuncture	Watertown, MA
Northwest Institute of Acupuncture and Oriental Medicine	Seattle, WA
Oregon College of Oriental Medicine	Portland, OR
Pacific College of Oriental Medicine	San Diego, CA
Samra University of Oriental Medicine	Los Angeles, CA
Santa Barbara College of Oriental Medicine	Santa Barbara, CA
Southwest Acupuncture College	Santa Fe, NM
Texas College of Traditional Chinese Medicine	Austin, TX
Yo Sa University of Traditional Chinese Medicine	Santa Monica, CA

SCHOOLS OF ASIAN MEDICINE AND ACUPUNCTURE

As part of their endeavor to professionalize themselves, acupuncturists have established training institutions around the United States. Acupuncture tends to be taught in schools of East Asian medicine. Indeed, the Office of Alternative Medicine reports that many American schools of acupuncture have developed into "colleges of Oriental medicine" by adding courses in Oriental massage, herbalism, and dietary therapy (1992:71). There are more than 50 schools of acupuncture and Oriental Medicine in the United States (see table 3). According to Grossinger, the American College of Traditional Chinese Medicine in San Francisco "has a tough medical-school level program in many holistic disciplines" (1990:404). The rigor of training at the many other acupuncture or East Asian medical schools is difficult to assess.

NATUROPATHY, ACUPUNCTURE, AND THE HOLISTIC HEALTH MOVEMENT

Both the rejuvenation of naturopathy and the emergence of acupuncture occurred within the context of the holistic health movement, which developed in the early 1970s, particularly on the West Coast. This movement, which I discuss in greater detail in the following chapter, drew from a number of contemporaneous movements and trends, particularly the hippie counterculture of the late 1960s and humanistic psychology. In *Making of a Counter Culture,* Theodore Roszak (1969) questioned the legitimacy claimed by biomedicine. The hippie counterculture sought health care that was compatible with its values of egalitarianism, naturalness, mysticism, "back to the land" philosophy, and vegetarianism. The "free clinic" movement of the 1960s and 1970s embodied many of these values. Like the counterculture, humanistic psychology rejected a technocratic and materialistic society and emphasized self-actualization and wholeness of body and mind. According to Berliner and Salmon, "though largely an outgrowth of the counterculture and human potential movements of the late 1960s and early 1970s, this [holistic health] movement has also been influenced strongly by current Chinese medical practices, Eastern philosophy, and nineteenth-century Western health practices" (1980:133). Alster, too, described the holistic health movement as a syncretic ensemble of the "mystical, the traditional, the occult, the Oriental, and common sense" (1989:44). Concurrent with these trends, a growing portion of the general public experienced general disenchantment with the high cost, bureaucratization, specialization, and reductionism of biomedicine. Many of these people were predisposed to the concepts and values of the holistic health movement.

Like the contemporary holistic health movement, naturopathy has since its beginnings been characterized by eclecticism. Benedict Lust, whom many consider to have been the father of American naturopathy, defined naturopathy as the "art of natural healing and of the science of physical and mental regeneration on the basis of self-reform, natural life, clean and normal diet, hydropathy, osteopathy, chiropractic, naturopathy, electrotherapy, diet, physiotherapy, physical and mental culture to the exclusion of poisonous drugs and non-adjustable surgery" (Fishbein 1932:125). Clivet C. Kristof, president of the North American Naturopathic Institute, stated, "We are the eclectics of the drugless healer. We use all methods" (quoted in Kruger 1974:182). Roth describes naturopaths as "out-and-out eclectics, using a great variety of esoteric herbs and other substances (which they prefer not to call drugs or medicine), shortwave heat treatments, exercises, and just about every other kind of therapy that has ever been developed" (1976:41).

The theoretical vagueness of naturopathy has enabled it to adjust to different health fads over the course of the twentieth century. Today, it incorporates homeopathy, Asian medical systems (such as acupuncture and Ayurveda), Evangelical faith healing, and New Age medicine. Because of its eclecticism, it was preadapted to the holistic health movement. As Rosch and Kearney observe, "holistic medicine relies upon the utilization of naturopathic modalities of therapy rather than upon pharmacologic agents or other artificial interventions" (1985:1407). Like other holistic health modalities, naturopathy emphasizes intuitive knowledge. Fuller's (1989:108) contention that the holistic health movement acted as a stimulant for the emergence of various New Age religions can be equally applied to naturopathy. According to Turner, naturopathy "underpins nearly all the therapeutic techniques in alternative medicine" (1984:25). Many naturopathic students identify with the countercultural movements, and some adhere to a form of Evangelical Protestantism that stresses healthful living and eating. Furthermore, as Roth demonstrates, the environmental, consumer rights, and hippie movements have given "natural healers" a wider audience than they had in the past (1976:122–24).

R. A. Dale implicitly proclaimed the embeddedness of American acupuncture in the holistic health movement at the founding convention of the American Association of Acupuncturists and Oriental Medicine in Los Angeles in 1981:

> Acupuncture is a part of a larger struggle going on today between the old and new, between dying and rebirthing, between the very decay and death of our species and our fullest liberation. Acupuncture is part of a New Age which facilitates integral health and flowering of our humanity. (quoted in Skrabanek 1985: 191)

Dale delineated five responses of biomedical practitioners toward acupuncture: "reactionary extreme," "conservative opposition," "liberal support," "progressive support," and "medical heretics." It appears that medical acupuncturists are divided, as Saks observes, into a "majority group who wish to restrict acupuncture to a limited range of applications within orthodox neurophysiological thinking and a minority who are more sympathetic to classical theories of acupuncture and wish to apply the technique to a broader span of maladies" (1995:174). Practitioners adopting the latter position probably tend to identify themselves as holistic medical physicians. In his address, Dale urged acupuncturists to present themselves to the public as acupuncture generalists rather than as medical specialists.

SOCIAL PROFILES OF NATUROPATHS AND ACUPUNCTURISTS

Far less research has been done on the social profile of naturopaths and acupuncturists than on that of chiropractors. In an interview, Ann Mitchell, N.D., stated that there are three generations of naturopaths: "old-school naturopaths trained in basic naturopathic techniques and principles in the 1920s; those trained in chiropractic who have a naturopathic interest; and those who have graduated in the past few years with rigorous science backgrounds from the two contemporary schools [NCNM and JBCNM]" (Finken 1986:43). The

Table 4   Profile of Students at John Bastyr College of Naturopathic Medicine

Entering Class	1982	1983	1984	1985	1986
Number	31	41	35	36	31
Average Age	28.4	29.0	29.5	29.3	30.0
Sex					
Female	11	19	16	17	22
Male	20	22	19	19	9
Undergraduate Degree	22	26	26	26	22
Graduate Degree	10	6	4	3	1

Source: Adapted from *Self-Study for Preparation of the Northwest Association of Schools and Colleges,* John Bastyr College of Naturopathic Medicine

profile of students at JBCNM (see table 4) appears to be somewhat different from that of students at biomedical schools. A social profile of freshmen biomedical students conducted at Duke University, the University of North Carolina, and the Bowman Gray School of Medicine indicated that 5.89 percent, 36.2 percent, and 18.3 percent, respectively, of the students at these three institutions were 24 years of age or older and that 31.5 percent, 22.0 percent, and 25.0 percent, respectively, were women (Leserman 1981:81). A survey showed that 38.2 percent of the 1989–1990 entering class at all biomedical schools and 36.1 percent of all students were women (Jonas, Etzel, and Barzansky 1990:804). While statistics on the average age of current biomedical students are difficult to obtain, it appears that it has been increasing somewhat due to a growing tendency on the part of biomedical schools to admit a greater number of "nontraditional" students. According to the Office of Admissions at the University of Arkansas for Medical Sciences, most of the 150 entering students in the 1989–1990 academic year were between 21 and 25 years of age, but ten were 35 years of age or older. While most JBCNM students have earned an undergraduate degree, it is generally one in pre-medicine or a biological science. On average, naturopathic students tend to be several years older than biomedical ones. Except for the entering class of 1982, the sex ratio at JBCNM differs appreciably from that at biomedical schools; female naturopaths, who established Women in Naturopathy (WIN) in 1987, have made up a high percentage of students graduating from JBCNM.

Although initially many nonbiomedical acupuncturists in the United States were of Asian extraction, more and more of them now appear to be of Anglo-American extraction. According to Anderson, all of the clinical instructors at the American College of Traditional Chinese Medicine in the early 1990s were immigrants who had obtained training in China, but most of the students were Americans who were not of Chinese descent (1991:463). The school also had some foreign students, particularly from Europe, Latin America, and Israel. Due to the low representation of Asian or Asian American students in

American acupuncture schools of Asian medicine, Asian acupuncturists have become a "distinct minority" within acupuncture (Kao and McRae 1990:270).

THE FUTURE OF NATUROPATHY AND ACUPUNCTURE AS PROFESSIONALIZED HETERODOX MEDICAL SYSTEMS

The future of both naturopathy and acupuncture in the United States remains tenuous. Twaddle and Hessler maintain that naturopathy is currently in a "state of ferment," particularly concerning issues such as the curricula of its colleges, the definition of its scope of practice, the distinction between itself and biomedicine, and the threat of biomedicine's incorporation of naturopathic therapies (1987:189). The Pacific Northwest continues to provide the most favorable sociopolitical climate for naturopaths. The American Holistic Medical Association has its headquarters in Seattle. While graduates of Bastyr University and the NCNM have been establishing practices in other states, such as Arizona, Florida, Texas, Connecticut, and Michigan, the growth of American naturopathy will remain restricted for some time to come because of the paucity of four-year schools. Acupuncture, with its more geographically far-flung network of schools, may already have come to supersede naturopathy as a professionalized heterodox medical system.

Unlike chiropractic, which no longer poses a serious threat to biomedicine because of its status as a specialty emphasizing spinal manipulation, a rejuvenated naturopathy finds itself in direct competition with biomedicine because both systems claim to provide a comprehensive approach to health care. Naturopaths utilizing spinal manipulation also face potential turf battles with chiropractors and even with osteopathic physicians specializing in manipulative therapy. Acupuncture also poses increasing competition for biomedicine as well as for chiropractic and naturopathy because it, too, defines itself as a form of comprehensive primary care. Indeed, Anderson asserts that acupuncturists as well as herbalists "are encroaching in part on chiropractic territory, in part on an area of competence claimed by a wide variety of mental health professionals, and in part on the domain of family practitioners" (1991:466).

As osteopathy and chiropractic did earlier, naturopathy and acupuncture are increasingly incorporating the theory and social organization of biomedicine. In preparing students to pass state licensing requirements, naturopathic and acupuncture schools modified their curricula to include extensive training in the basic sciences. Emulating the tendency toward specialization in biomedicine, an increasing number of naturopaths focus on modalities such as acupuncture, homeopathy, psychological medicine, obstetrics, and manipulation. Some AANP members belong to the Naturopathic Physicians Acupuncture Association (American Association of Naturopathic Physicians 3[5] 1988).

In theory, naturopathy and acupuncture, like the larger holistic health movement, contain the potential to serve as part of what Lyng (1990) terms a "medical countersystem." According to McKee, "the naturopathic view of illness as a process or activity initiated by the body in adaptive response to an unnatural environment challenges the Western view of disease as malfunction, as an entity—as something that happens to the individual as a consequence of assault by an external agent" (1988:778). In reality, however, both naturopaths and acupuncturists, like most biomedical physicians, tend to ignore the economic, political, and social origins of diseases and to focus on individual rather than societal responsibility for health maintenance. Along with an increasing number of biomedical physicians, naturopaths point to lifestyle factors as the source of disease. McKee maintains that naturopathy, like other holistic therapies, adheres to the

> individualist philosophy which prevails in capitalism. The environmental conditions . . . which naturopathic and other holistic treatment is directed to correct are the inner (physical, psychological, and spiritual), rather than outer, social influences. (1988:778)

Both naturopathy and acupuncture, with their reductionist philosophies and their focus on individual responsibility for healthy living, may well undergo further growth during an era of growing health costs.

6

Partially Professionalized and Lay Heterodox Medical Systems within the Context of the Holistic Health Movement

European American partially professionalized and lay heterodox medical systems existed within the context of two health movements during the twentieth century. The first one has been called the "natural health movement" by Roth (1976), who views it as a continuation of the health reform movement of the nineteenth century, discussed in chapter 1. The second one is the holistic health/New Age movement, which I mentioned in the previous chapter and discuss in more detail in this chapter. Both of these movements have contained within them a variety of professionalized heterodox practitioners as well as some biomedical practitioners. Around the early 1970s, a certain amount of overlap developed between the two movements, with the latter in large part incorporating the former and moving beyond it. Certain lay therapists within both movements have made some attempts to professionalize, but others have resisted it. In commenting upon this resistance, Pizer notes that "many of the new practitioners are extremely individualistic in their philosophy and lifestyle, and resent professional control of any form" (1982:188).

THE NATURAL HEALTH MOVEMENT AS A PRECURSOR OF THE HOLISTIC HEALTH MOVEMENT

The natural health movement was a diverse phenomenon developed by "health purifiers," or "natural healthers," to address the impacts of air and water pollution and food additives on health. Bernarr Macfadden appears to have served as a transitional figure between the health reform movement of the nineteenth century and the natural health movement that emerged in the early twentieth century. In an effort to overcome his weak constitution during adolescence, Macfadden strengthened himself by lifting dumbbells and walking long distances. Macfadden referred to his health prevention system as Physical Culture and in 1899 began to publish *Physical Culture*, a magazine that made him a multimillionaire. According to Whorton,

His pen and presses were also responsible for a gamut of health handbooks stretching from *Hair Culture* through *Strengthening the Spine* to *Foot Troubles* and many, many others. His *Encyclopedia of Physical Culture* gave a five-volume exposition of the system practiced at his several Physical Culture "Healthatoriums" . . . . Macfadden's system, also called "Physcultopathy," was largely a modernized version of Jacksonian health reform, its blend of unstimulating diet, exercise, sunshine and fresh air, cleanliness, and no medicine being rationalized by subjective interpretations of contemporary biological science. (1982:297)

Sociologist Julius A. Roth identified six categories of "services and institutions" that assisted "natural healthers" in their search for health: "(1) natural health practitioners, (2) natural health hospitals or health resorts, (3) health food stores and merchant organizations, (4) natural health nutritionists, (5) protective organizations, and (6) publicity (or education) [through] lecturers, magazines, [and] books (often published by special houses)" (1976:13). Natural healthers viewed Big Business as the source of much pollution, and Big Government, especially regulatory agencies, as serving to protect industry's polluting practices. They regarded the Food and Drug Administration as a major culprit in this regard for failing to control the pharmaceutical industry and food manufacturers and for requiring prescriptions for natural food supplements, thus cutting into a source of profit for health food stores (Roth 1976:9–10).

Natural health practitioners consisted primarily of two types of therapists: naturopathic practitioners and natural hygienists. Naturopathic practitioners included within their ranks naturopaths, chiropractors, osteopaths, homeopaths with M.D.s, naprapaths, and "naturalized" M.D.s (biomedical physicians who had adopted natural health methods), as well as therapists who employed herbalism, acupuncture, concept therapy, and wheat grass therapy. They tended to be rather eclectic and prescribed a wide variety of treatment modalities for their patients. As noted in the previous chapter, many naturopathic practitioners viewed themselves as professionals and sought to achieve recognition as such. In contrast, natural hygienists tended to eschew professionalization and generally did not have training institutions or licenses of their own, although some of them felt that it might be wise to strive for these forms of legitimation. Many natural hygienists were converted chiropractors or naturopaths. Whereas naturopathic practitioners were pragmatists willing to make compromises with what they considered the "polluting" habits of the larger society, natural hygienists were the ultimate purists who viewed medical practices such as immunization as unnatural forms of poisoning the body. They tended to conduct their practices at resorts rather than in offices.

Roth (1976:98–99) maintains that clients tended to be recruited into the natural health movement through health food stores, health magazines, natural health organization meetings, and health resorts. He notes,

> The mecca of such institutions and of the Natural Hygiene world is Shelton's Health School. The founder, Herbert Shelton, is Natural Hygiene's leading spokesman and his prolific writings have covered just about every conceivable health issue. . . . The health school is considered by many in the movement as the purest expression of the Natural Hygiene life style because of the congruence of Natural Hygiene ideology and practices of the health school. The diet is largely raw fruit and vegetables and nuts with minimal cutting, shredding, and juicing. (1976:19)

Gaylord Hauser, another prominent natural hygienist, promoted diets low in meat and high in organic fruits and vegetables from the 1920s to the 1950s and reportedly made salads a popular component of Southern California cuisine (Goldstein 1992:57). Adele Davis, the author of numerous nutritional guides, argued that "adoption of her dietary ideas would lead to greater emotional and spiritual health, world peace, courage, integrity, and love" (Goldstein 1992: 58).

The National Health Federation (NHF) served as an umbrella group for many natural healthers. Founded in 1955 by Fred J. Hart, president of the Electronic Medical Foundation, NHF calls for "freedom of choice" by health consumers. The NHF claims that it neither opposes nor approves any specific medical system, but it does oppose the efforts of any health care profession to create a medical monopoly: each issue of its monthly *Bulletin* states that it "opposes monopoly and compulsion in things related to health where the safety and welfare of others are not concerned" (quoted in Barrett 1976:195). The NHF board has included food supplement and vitamin manufacturers, owners of natural stores, chiropractors, naturopaths, and other types of practitioners. The organization "gives legal aid to persons prosecuted for supposed violations of restrictions on health activities; lobbies to expand the scope of practice for unorthodox healing arts; [and] opposes compulsory programs of fluoridation, vaccination, and pasteurization" (Roth 1976:28). Whereas the NHF was initially run mostly by political ultraconservatives, by the 1970s its leadership came to consist of more moderate voices who were concerned about achieving some semblance of legitimacy in the larger society.

The natural health movement was transformed in the 1960s and 1970s, in part as a result of the interest of counterculturalists in "natural" living issues. Roth observes:

> The advent of hippies on the natural scene has produced a dilemma for some of the founding fathers of the natural health movement in the United States. . . . On the one hand, the old-timers should be delighted to find their hard-fought campaign bearing fruit in an increasing number of adherents, especially from the oncoming generation. At the same time, they were shocked by their association with these obviously immoral and subversive beings. (1976:32–33)

105

In contrast to the rather accommodating posture of the NHF, the American Natural Hygiene Society adopted a more hard-line stance on health practices. The society was established by Shelton in 1948 and opposes compulsory immunization, fluoridation, and food irradiation (Zwicky et al. 1993). Roth characterizes it as "primarily an organization of lay adherents and publicists in which the few practitioners have a special consultative role, but are not a controlling force" (1976:28). On its Web site, the society claims that it has over 10,000 members in 50 countries. It asserts that natural hygiene is a "philosophy and a set of principles and practices based on science that lead to an extraordinary level of personal health and happiness." The society advocates vegetarianism, with an emphasis on large amounts of fresh fruits, nuts, and either uncooked or steamed vegetables, and a lifestyle that incorporates plenty of rest, sleep, exercise, fresh air, sunshine, and pure distilled water.

The more pragmatic adherents of the natural health movement came to form a loose alliance with consumer advocates, environmentalists, and advocates of alternative lifestyles. Concerns about nutrition, wellness, and the environment are no longer fringe activities monopolized by ultraconservatives opposed to government welfare programs, public schools, and "creeping socialism." Instead, these have become avant-garde issues that interest a wide array of relatively well-educated people, including political liberals and radicals, yuppies, and New Agers.

THE HOLISTIC HEALTH MOVEMENT
AS A MASS PHENOMENON

Although the natural health movement per se has not completely passed from the scene, much of its thunder has been stolen by the holistic health movement. The holistic health movement encompasses an extremely varied assortment of alternative medical therapies and practices. It encompasses aspects of humanistic and psychosomatic medicine, parapsychology, folk medicine, herbalism, nutritional therapies, homeopathy, yoga, massage and other forms of bodywork, meditation, and the martial arts (Berliner and Salmon 1979, 1980). Its diverse cast of characters includes lay alternative practitioners, psychic or spiritual healers, New Agers, holistic M.D.s, and at least some osteopathic physicians, chiropractors, naturopaths, and acupuncturists. As noted in the previous chapter, the holistic health movement grew out of several other movements, particularly the counterculture of the late 1960s with its emphasis on "getting back to nature" and disenchantment with mainstream culture and institutions, the human potential movement, Eastern philosophy and medicine, and nineteenth-century Western heterodox medical systems (e.g., homeopathy, osteopathy, chiropractic, and naturopathy). The counterculture, a major stimulus of the holistic health movement, drew upon a wide array of psychotherapies, including Werner Erhard's Seminar Training or est, Arica, bioenergetics, Silva Mind Control, Insight, primal therapy, and rebirthing. The establishment of the American Holistic Medical Association (AMHA) in 1978 indicated the growing interest of biomedical and osteopathic physicians in this popular health movement.

The holistic health movement has several well-known public spokespersons, including Norman Cousins, Bernie S. Siegel, Dolores Krieger, and Ken Pelletier. In his best-selling *Anatomy of Illness* (1979), Cousins, a former editor of *Saturday Review,* described how, through a regimen of optimistic and cheerful thinking, he overcame a serious disease for which biomedical physicians had given him a bleak prognosis. Bernie S. Siegel, a biomedical physician and health writer, encouraged cancer patients to read books on meditation and psychic phenomena in order to tap into higher healing energies. Ken Pelletier, a psychologist at the University of California, San Francisco, has written *Mind as Healer, Mind as Slayer* (1977), *Toward a Science of Consciousness* (1978), and *Holistic Medicine* (1979). Holistically oriented practitioners, including M.D.s, have established a number of magazines and journals, including the *Journal of Holistic Health, Alternative Medicine,* the *Holistic Health Review* (published by the American Holistic Medical Association), and the *Journal of Alternative and Complementary Medicine: Research on Paradigm, Practice, and Policy.*

The holistic health movement overlaps considerably with the New Age movement. As Melton et al. observe, the "New Age and Holistic Health movements in theory exist independently, but are united philosophically by one central concept: that the individual person is responsible for his or her own life and for seeking out the means of transformation needed to achieve a better quality of life" (1991:169). New Agers are staunch critics of the technological and depersonalized nature of Western society. They often view the holistic health movement as an integral part of their movement. The New Age movement seeks to create a "new planetary culture" that emphasizes inner tranquility, wellness, harmony, unity, self-realization, self-actualization, and the attainment of a higher level of consciousness (Grossinger 1990). Levin and Coreil (1986:894–95) delineate three New Age healing approaches: (1) body-oriented ones that emphasize the achievement of somatic and psychosomatic health, (2) mind-oriented ones that emphasize esoteric teachings as a mechanism for achieving health, and (3) soul-oriented ones that emphasize meditation and other contemplative techniques. New Age healing incorporates many therapeutic techniques and practices, including "centering, channeling, astral projection, guided visualization, iridology, reflexology, chromotherapy, rebirthing, shiatsu, and healing with the power of pyramids and crystals" (Danforth 1989:253). In *The Aquarian Conspiracy* (1980), one of the bibles of the New Age movement, Marilyn Ferguson espouses social transformation through personal transformation. She maintains that spiritual and holistic health practices will bring about a paradigm shift which in turn will contribute to the transformation of social institutions. Hess suggests that New Agers are "heirs to the side of the sixties counterculture that opted for spiritual transformation rather than direct social change" (1993:5).

Some New Agers define themselves as neopagans, who tend to view themselves as the victims of biomedicine. According to Orion, "almost every Neopagan thinks of him- or herself as a healer" (1995:182). Indeed, many neopagans define themselves as "shamans" or "shaman witches." Of the 189 neopagans in Orion's survey, 75.6 percent reported relying upon meditation, 73.0 percent upon visualization, 53.9 percent upon massage, 53.9 upon herbalism, 50.8 upon vitamin therapy, and 40.7 upon crystal therapy (Orion 1995:183). Some, if not many, neopagans use chiropractic, massage therapy, homeopathy, acupuncture, and various other alternative therapies. Michael York (1995: 33) argues that both the New Age movement and neopaganism are "manifestations of the Western occult tradition—specifically, of what is often termed the American metaphysical tradition"—a phenomenon that I discuss in the next chapter.

Many New Agers are proponents of neoshamanism, a movement that idealizes the shamanistic practices of Native Americans and other indigenous peoples around the globe. As Atkinson observes, "widespread popular interest in shamanism and multiculturalism has created a market for anthologies and recordings of shamans' narratives, songs, and other verbal genres" (1992: 320). Anthropologist Michael Harner, a former professor at the New School for Social Research, has become a New Age guru as a result of his popular book *The Way of the Shaman* (1990) and his creation of the Foundation for Shamanic Studies. He became intimately acquainted with shamanism among the Jivaro and Conibo Indians of South America and has developed a synthesis of universal shamanic practices, called "core shamanism," which he teaches in workshops around the country. On its Web site, the Dance of the Deer Foundation (est. 1979), based in the Santa Cruz Mountains of California, advertises its commitment to maintaining the shamanic traditions of the Huichol Indians of northern Mexico through seminars, pilgrimages, and study groups in the United States, Mexico, Europe, and other parts of the world. Some Native Americans, however, regard New Age dabbling into shamanism as an illegitimate appropriation of their cultures. In early 1994, the National Congress of American Indians declared war on "non-Indian 'wannabes,' hucksters, cultists, commercial profiteers and self-styled New Age shamans" (quoted in Glass-Coffin 1994:A48) for exploiting, distorting, and abusing American Indian religious traditions.

The holistic health movement and New Age healing first emerged on the

West Coast of the United States and then spread to other parts of this country, western Europe, and many other countries. Many New Age healing groups were first formed in the San Francisco Bay Area, the major center of the holistic health/New Age movement (Danforth 1989:252–53). The holistic health movement also has many other centers throughout the West Coast, such as Seattle and Portland. On the East Coast, centers include Greenwich Village and the East Village in Manhattan and Burlington, Vermont. Several inland cities and towns (such as Santa Fe, New Mexico; Sedona, Arizona; and Boulder, Colorado) have also emerged as New Age centers. Major institutions of the holistic health/New Age movement include the Holistic Health and Nutrition Institute in Mill Valley, California; the Open Education Exchange in Oakland; the East West Academy of Healing Arts in San Francisco; the Holistic Life University in San Francisco; the Southwest School of Botanical Medicine in Bisbee, Arizona; the Himalayan Institute (est. 1971) in the Pocono Mountains of northeastern Pennsylvania; the Yes Educational Society in Washington, D.C.; the Omega Institute in the Catskill Mountains of New York State; and the New York Open Center. Numerous holistic health centers employing teams consisting of biomedical physicians, chiropractors, naturopaths, psychologists, and other types of therapists have sprung up in many parts of the United States (Gordon 1984). Organizations emphasizing holistic health include the American Holistic Medical Association (est. 1978); the Association for Holistic Health, based in San Diego; Medical Holistics, based in Fresno, California; and the American Holistic Nurses Association, based in Raleigh, North Carolina.

The holistic health movement has become a mass phenomenon as a result of widespread dissatisfaction with the bureaucratic and iatrogenic aspects of biomedicine. Health food stores have played a central role in disseminating information about alternative therapies to a wider public during both the natural health movement and the holistic health movement. As Hufford and Chilton observe,

> In the United States, the health food movement has had the greatest influence in developing and disseminating natural healing ideas throughout the twentieth century. It has provided for an accessible model within which herbalism, nutritional therapy, environmental protection, a variety of lifestyle factors, including exercise, and spiritual concerns could be integrated and explored. Today the widespread availability of health food stores and the appearance of health food language in supermarkets both reflect and continue to advance public attention to natural healing ideas. (1996:64)

Figure 2 delineates many, but by no means all, of the partially professionalized and lay heterodox therapies or medical systems that have become incorporated within the larger rubric of the holistic health/New Age movement.

109

Figure 2   Selected Partially and Lay Heterodox Therapeutic Systems

Homeopathy
Herbalism
Bodywork
    Massage
    Rolfing
    Reflexology
    Acupressure
    Shiatsu
    Reiki
    Alexander Technique
    Feldenkreis Method
    Applied Kinesiology
Body/Mind Medicine
    Meditation
    Yoga
    Guided Visualization
    Biofeedback
    Bioenergetics
    Hypnotherapy
    Polarity Therapy
    Iridology
Lay Midwifery

THREE SOCIAL SETTINGS EMPHASIZING
HOLISTIC/NEW AGE HEALING PRACTICES

To date, only four in-depth ethnographic studies have been conducted on holistic/New Age healing practices in American society. The first of these was conducted by Craig Molgaard (1979, 1981) on a healing commune he called Agni Circle (pseudonym) in north central Washington State. In the second, Loring M. Danforth (1989) focused on firewalking as a New Age healing ritual. J. A. English-Lueck (1990) studied New Age practitioners, workshops, and institutions over a two-year period in a small Southern California coastal city (pop. 75,000) he called Paraiso (pseudonym). I discuss the fourth, June S. Lowenberg's (1989) study of a holistic health center in California, in the concluding chapter because its two primary practitioners were biomedical physicians rather than partially or lay heterodox practitioners.

AGNI CIRCLE

Agni Circle was established in 1976 in a town of some 800 people near a large lake. It consisted of nine men, seven women, and three children. About half of its members lived in a post office building on the town's Main Street, and the others resided in scattered houses in the town or in small cabins in nearby apple orchards. Agni Circle conducted healing services and classes on massage, yoga, anatomy, and astrology and provided treatment to anyone who desired it, generally migrant or seasonal New Age agricultural workers. The commune also operated an alternative recreational center for agricultural workers and conducted an annual healing gathering in the spring that attracted up to 900 people. Women tended to be the "therapeutic innovators," with men following their lead in the use of various therapies. Philosophically, Agni Circle's members blended together a "superficially confusing array of Ayurvedic, Chinese, native American, chiropractic, and homeopathic beliefs" (Molgaard 1981:157).

The commune's healers relied primarily upon massage, Bach flower therapy, lithotherapy, and herbalism. Bach flower therapy is a homeopathic remedy that is intended to restore spiritual and emotional harmony. Lithotherapy relies upon stones and gems to ward off negative energy vibrations and also pendulum crystals to stimulate energy flow. Although women functioned as the primary healers at Agni Circle, the men served as the commune's elders. Patients sought treatment for ailments ranging from epilepsy to severe burns to staph infections. Agni Circle was part of a network of healing communes in the Pacific Northwest. Ironically, the most famous healers among them tended to be males, for example, Jeff, in Spokane, an iridologist; Michael, in Vancouver, who specialized in energy treatments; and Jack Bond, of Oregon, who specialized in kinesiology. Like Agni Circle, other healing communes also conducted annual healing gatherings. These gatherings functioned as a mechanism for exchanging information about therapeutic lore and providing New Age people with a "sense of belonging to a larger whole" (Molgaard 1979:59).

NEW AGE FIREWALKING

In New Age firewalking, participants test their level of self-realization by walking barefoot on hot coals at nighttime, outdoor celebrations. Tolly Burkan is considered to be the founding father of American firewalking and has lectured at the University of Arizona Medical Center and the Mandalla Growth Center in Oslo, Norway (Danforth 1989:260). In 1977 he incorporated firewalking into his workshops on self-awareness, spiritual transformation, and personal growth. In 1982 Burkan and his wife "developed a four-hour walking workshop designed to help people overcome their fears and limitations because they realized that 'the firewalk was the perfect metaphor to encompass all aspects of life'" (Danforth 1989:261). According to Ken Cardigan, a prominent firewalker whose full-moon firedance celebration Danforth (1989: 222) attended in the Maine woods, firewalking constitutes an empowering ritual that adherents believe can produce both physiological healing, even for cancer patients, and psychological healing.

Anthony Robbins is the other nationally renowned leader of American fire-walking. He founded the Robbins Research Institute and has served as a consultant for Olympic athletes, the United States Army, and corporate executives:

> One of Robbins's most publicized seminars was held at Hilton Head, South Carolina, in September 1985, as part of the annual convention of Record Bar, Inc., the second largest retailer of records and tapes in the United States. The seminar, for which Robbins received seventy-five thousand dollars, was part of the company's "human systems" program in developing its workers' potential to the fullest. (Danforth 1989:263)

PARAISO: A CALIFORNIA HOLISTIC/NEW AGE HEALING CENTER

Paraiso, the pseudonymous town studied by English-Lueck (1990), was made up largely of white upper-middle- and upper-class residents but also had small enclaves of Chicanos (10 percent), Asians (2 percent), and Native Americans (nearly 1 percent). Despite this relative ethnic homogeneity, Paraiso's residents followed a variety of lifestyles: there were millionaires who tended to live in the city's higher elevations, university students, street people, "resident vagabonds," and members of "non-conventional" religious groups, such as the Unitarian-Universalist Church, the Unity School of Christianity, and the Church of Religious Science. In addition to health food restaurants, imported natural clothing boutiques, alternative New Age craft shops, and exercise centers, it had numerous self-help groups and 36 schools that offered workshops and lectures on alternative medicine. School A certified its graduates as "holistic health practitioners" and offered credentials in massage and hypnosis as well as continuing education for nurses. School B trained massage therapists, and School C trained acupuncturists. Workshops on alternative therapies were offered at the local community college, a university extension program, the YMCA, herbal stores, a Taoist sanctuary, and a Yogic Institute/ashram.

Three types of alternative or heterodox practitioners had been present in Paraiso at one time or other: (1) "renowned catalysts," or founders of well-known therapies who either visited the community or resided there, (2) "publicly visible practitioners," who generally also functioned as teachers, and (3) novice practitioners. Of the estimated 790 to 830 heterodox practitioners in the Paraiso area, only 253 practiced publicly. Many certified practitioners did not advertise, preferring to function within small, intimate networks to avoid legal harassment. Heterodox practitioners often were therapeutically eclectic, combining different therapies depending upon the needs and desires of the patient. Bodyworkers incorporated approaches such as massage, yoga, Alexander technique, and reflexology or zone therapy into their practices. Clients found practitioners through both public and private networks. Some "regulars" had appointments as often as once a week, and others made one or two visits to a practitioner and then moved on to a new one. In its diversity of practitioners, Paraiso constitutes something of a microcosm of the holistic health movement.

THE DRIVE FOR PROFESSIONALIZATION AMONG LAY HETERODOX PRACTITIONERS

A drive for professionalization has appeared repeatedly among heterodox practitioners, in the sense that many have sought to obtain legitimacy, generally in the form of licensing or certification from the state or recognition from an accrediting body, even one internal to a specific alternative medical system. English-Lueck (1990:155–58) identified four steps in the process by which heterodox practitioners in Paraiso and elsewhere undergo professionalization: (1) full-time activity as a healer or therapist; (2) establishment of a school or accredited academy; (3) establishment of an association, such as the American Massage Therapy Association; and (4) establishment of an umbrella organization, such as the California Health Practitioners Association.

Homeopathy is one of the main heterodox medical systems that has been undergoing professionalization. Health practitioners of various types have been attempting to rejuvenate and reprofessionalize homeopathy, which had lost the professional status it held in the nineteenth century, within the context of the holistic health movement. Homeopathy first captured the interest of certain biomedical students who were seeking therapeutic alternatives during the turbulent 1960s. According to Coulter, "there are several hundred allopathically trained physicians practicing homoeopathy exclusively as well as several thousand who use it occasionally, not to mention the many nurses, osteopaths, chiropractors, veterinarians, clinical psychologists, and naturopathic practitioners who also employ homoeopathy" (1984:73). Connecticut, Arizona, Nevada, and Washington are the only states that license homeopaths (Studdert et al. 1998:1614). Apparently, numerous lay heterodox practitioners employ homeopathic medicines because of their nonprescription status in the United States. Borre and Wilson (1998:83) maintain that homeopathy is a part of consumers' takeover of their own health care. Many retail drug and food stores now sell homeopathic remedies, and advertisements for them appear regularly on national television and in popular magazines. The public

113

and biomedical physicians have expressed a growing interest in enrolling in homeopathic courses and study groups.

In the late 1970s, the San Francisco Bay Area reportedly became "the center of a new revival of homeopathy led largely by nonphysicians" (Gurin 1979: 12). In April 1978 George Vithoulkas, a world-renowned homeopathic physician from Greece, gave 15 hours of lectures to an assemblage of some 500 people at the California Academy of Sciences in San Francisco. Grossinger reports:

> For the older homeopaths there, it must have been a both deeply disturbing and elating event. . . . M.D.s had their hair in braids and wore turbans and robes, and country enthusiasts came down from parts of Oregon, Idaho, Washington, Nevada, Utah, New Mexico, California, etc., dressed for the road or the farm, bearded and long-haired. . . . the American Institute of Homeopathy fears that an awakening of this sort will bring down the wrath of the AMA and the Food and Drug Administration (FDA), which, to this point, have been content to let homeopathy quietly die out without challenging the older practitioners. (1990: 242)

The conference prompted the establishment of the International Foundation for the Promotion of Homeopathy. Vithoulkas "spoke of both the enthusiasm and the superficiality of the new homeopathy . . . . [and] announced that he would no longer receive lay practitioners at his seminar in Athens" (Grossinger 1990:241–42).

David Ullman, an East Bay–based layperson, has been a key player in the homeopathic revival. In 1976 he was indicted for allegedly having violated the California Medical Practice Act. Attorney Jerry Green "argued that because Ullman practiced a different form of healing, he should not have been considered as practicing medicine" (Pizer 1982:177). The state of California dropped its charges against Ullman, who holds a master's degree in public health and functions as a homeopathic educator, writing articles and books about homeopathy, serving as president of the Foundation of Homoeopathic Education and Research and director of Homoeopathic Educational Services, and lecturing and running workshops on homeopathy. Ullman contends that "since homeopathic medicines are known to be considerably safer than conventional drugs, their use in the 21st century will sharply reduce the amount of iatrogenic (doctor-induced) disease" (Ullman 1991).

Tensions between professionalists and counterculturalists run deep within the homeopathic revival—but the former appear to be coming out ahead. The Council on Homeopathic Education has accredited five programs: the National College of Naturopathic Medicine in Portland, Bastyr University of Natural Health Sciences in Seattle, Ontario College of Naturopathic Medicine in Toronto, Hahnemann Medical Clinic in Berkeley, and the International Foundation for Homeopathy in Seattle (Collinge 1996:162). Other homeopathic training programs include the Pacific Academy of Homeopathic Medicine in Berkeley and the New England School of Homeopathy in Amherst, Massachusetts. In contrast to the popular orientation of the Pacific Academy of Homeopathy in San Francisco, the Hahnemann College of Homeopathy and Medical College in Albany, an East Bay community, exemplifies the efforts of various homeopaths either to professionalize themselves or to further legitimize their endeavors, especially in instances where they already hold biomedical credentials (Vespucci 1994). The Hahnemann College offers courses only to licensed health professionals, such as M.D.s, nurse practitioners, acupuncturists, podiatrists, and veterinarians. It does not admit Ph.D. psychologists. Licensed health professionals who practice homeopathy in the United States are listed in a directory sold by the Homeopathic Educational Services and the National Center for Homeopathy, based in Berkeley (Ullman 1991). Grossinger contends that homeopathy is at a crossroads in the United States because it is being practiced again by "new professionals and is available to the public" (1990:243–44).

Homeopaths, whether physicians or nonphysicians, are not the only heterodox practitioners who are attempting to professionalize themselves. Hypnotherapists in California are attempting to increase their standards of certification by trying to eliminate weekend or short-course certification schools (McClendon 1994). Naturopathy has licensing laws in eleven states, including Oregon, Washington, and Alaska, but not California. Many California naturopaths practice under either an acupuncture or a chiropractic license. The California Association of Naturopathic Physicians (CANP), an affiliate of the American Association of Naturopathic Physicians, has been involved in a difficult campaign to obtain licensing for graduates of four-year naturopathic colleges. It has been attempting to restrict the activities of the graduates of short-term naturopathic schools, over 300 of whom are represented by the California Naturopathic Medical Association. Thus far, CANP has been very limited in its efforts because of the high costs of lobbying activities in the California legislature.

An increasing number of lay midwives have embarked upon a process of professionalization. The late 1960s and early 1970s witnessed not only a significant rise in nurse midwifery but also a resurgence of lay midwifery. The latter development was part and parcel of the countercultural home birth movement, which emerged within the context of the natural birth and holistic health/New Age movements. The Farm, a hippie commune started by Stephen Gaskin and his followers in middle Tennessee in the early 1970s, established a well-publicized lay midwifery program (Traugot 1998:46). Ina

May Gaskin, Stephen's wife, assumed the task of becoming community midwife and obtained advice from a local physician. The Farm published *Spiritual Midwifery*, a book that became very popular in lay midwifery circles.

Lay midwifery appealed to others besides hippies or countercultural people. Ironically, as Cobb observes, "at precisely the time when members of low income and rural populations have been persuaded to give up home births, certain segments of the white American middle class are seeking birth at home, and it is the home birth couples themselves and the modern lay midwife as well as selected physicians and nurse-midwives who have responded to this demand" (1981:82). Lay midwives formed a national organization, the Midwifery Alliance of North America (MANA), in 1982 (Bourgeault and Fynes 1997:1056). Despite lay midwives' initial suspicions about biomedicine, Reid suggests that the "continued pressure for licensure in major states like California suggests that [lay midwives] may well have accepted integration and domination as the viable option" (1989:238). Indeed, some lay midwives in California have welcomed efforts to license their occupation as a means to improve its quality and status (DeVries 1982:83). MANA representatives played a role in creating the North American Registry Examination for Midwives (NAREM) in 1991. An estimated 1,500 to 2,000 lay midwives were practicing in the United States in the mid-1990s (Bourgeault and Fynes 1997:1056). Because licensing will inevitably entail some degree of physician supervision, lay midwifery faces the danger of being co-opted by biomedicine, despite the fact that in large measure it emerged as a counter-hegemonic response to it. At the moment, the biomedical profession is more hostile to lay midwifery than to nurse midwifery. As a result of increasing numbers of malpractice suits and cost of malpractice insurance premiums, physicians are increasingly opting out of practicing obstetrics. Nurse midwives, but also lay midwives, have been filling a niche that many obstetricians have vacated. At the macroscopic level, the increasing corporatization of medicine in the United States may prompt insurance companies seeking inexpensive approaches to health care to be receptive to reimbursing partially professionalized or lay midwives (DeVries 1993:137).

Bodyworkers have established several certifying organizations. One of them, the American Massage Therapy Association (AMTA, est. 1943), which reportedly has over 18,000 members (Collinge 1996:300), is striving to professionalize Swedish massage. According to Mertz,

> AMTA standards for entry-level education specifies [sic] 500 hours of course work. As of 1994, its Commission on Massage Training and Accreditation/Approval (COMTAA) listed 59 schools throughout the US and Canada. . . . There are approximately 150 schools located in California, where the minimum hours required for certification to work in a health spa or chiropractor's office is 100.

In California, certification is granted by massage schools, and certified massage therapists (CMTs) with this minimal training have the choice of joining the Associated Bodywork and Massage Professionals (ABMP) or the International Massage Association (IMA) in order to acquire necessary liability insurance. (1996:3)

Massage therapy is regulated in a variety of ways in 22 of 50 states (Mertz 1996:7). In Maryland, the chiropractic board oversees licensing of massage therapists, whereas in Texas massage therapists are required to be registered with the Department of Health. The AMTA has been striving to establish itself as the primary professional organization for massage therapists, while the ABMP is attempting to organize practitioners of a variety of bodywork modalities.

Despite a tendency by many lay heterodox practitioners to seek professionalization, other practitioners strongly eschew this process. In the case of Paraiso, English-Lueck reports:

Some practitioners do not want to organize. The freedom that they experience, especially as lay practitioners, is what drew them to the movement. Joining organizations and becoming established is not what they sought. The individualism of the early Gnostics and the Theosophists created perpetual fission, thriving in informal networks of allies until a new vision comes along. Similarly, Doug—a pioneer in Paraiso's holistic health community—having rebelled against his establishment life, was resistant to professionalization. He wanted no "organic fascists" to interfere with his practice or his life-style. (1990:152)

Instead, such heterodox practitioners prefer to operate within a small pre-existing social network of friends and acquaintances who become clients or patients.

THE HOLISTIC HEALTH MOVEMENT: A CASE OF MEDICAL COUNTER-HEGEMONY OR HEGEMONY?

Berliner and Salmon (1979) argued that during its early stages, the holistic health movement contained the potential to pick up the banner of social medicine and function as a critique of capitalist institutions, despite its apolitical, entrepreneurial, elitist, and authoritarian tendencies. Lyng (1990) has described the holistic health movement as a "countersystem" that challenges, in part, biomedical hegemony. Melton et al. observe that "strains of anarchism, Marxism, libertarianism, corporate capitalism, pacifism, communitarianism, individualism, occultism, and romanticism coexist (albeit nervously)" within the New Age movement (1991:428). (What Melton et al. refer to as Marxism is more accurately described as a loosely defined mystical socialism.)

Some heterodox practitioners have been able to override opposition from biomedicine to their licensing or even to their provision of services in biomedical settings. Furthermore, the corporate class and its state sponsors may provide support to heterodox medical systems if they feel that these systems serve certain functions for them or are cheaper than biomedicine. As I have noted, various holistic health practitioners have made a concerted effort to develop a medical "countersystem" that resists processes of professionalization. Others have embarked upon a drive for professionalization that will ensure them a share of the medical marketplace. While these patterns of legitimation and even professionalization may illustrate, on the one hand, that indeed the dominance of organized biomedicine is limited, they reflect, on the other hand, a growing accommodation by heterodox practitioners, including those who fall under the rubric of the holistic health/New Age movement, to a reductionist theory compatible with capitalist ideology and to the biomedical model of organization and social control.

For the most part, the holistic health movement in its present form engages in a rather limited holism, in that its focus is largely on the individual rather than on society and its institutions (Alster 1989; Goldstein 1992). Holistic health practitioners tend to downplay occupational and environmental hazards, such as air and water pollution and toxic waste, because these are viewed as beyond the individual's immediate control. In emphasizing individual responsibility for health, the holistic health movement functions as an alternative form of medical hegemony by reinforcing individualizing patterns in American society. As Montgomery so astutely observes, "never in this [holistic health] discourse are there allotments [sic] made for such things as class, race, age, or the like" (1993:83).

Furthermore, the holistic health/New Age movement tends to downplay community service, social reform, and other collective goals. Danforth (1989: 260) maintains that the New Age movement legitimizes "utilitarian individualism" and a "materialist concern for upward social mobility" in the context of the countercultural ideology that its adherents learned during the 1960s. He asserts that despite their purported concern with social problems such as racism, poverty, and environmental degradation, New Agers "fail to realize that it requires more than personal growth and self-transformation to change long-standing public policies and powerful social institutions, nor do they realize that their idealistic and utopian visions for social change are doomed because they fail to take into account the oppressive aspects of the social, political, and economic order that are ultimately responsible for the problems of so many people" (Danforth 1989:284–85). In a similar vein, Ivakhiv observes in his overview of the New Age community in Sedona, Arizona, that "for all its mythologizing of the Sedona–Red Rock landscape, it is a rare event when the *Sedona Journal of Emergence* actually urges its readers to do some-

118

thing (in the 'third dimension' of physical and social reality) about some environmental issue" (1997:379).

Like biomedicine and certain established professionalized heterodox medical systems, particularly chiropractic, the holistic health/New Age movement shows signs of becoming increasingly entrepreneurial. Rosch and Kearney note that it has "witnessed the appearance of a number of entrepreneurs and even charlatans who seek to exploit the appeal of 'holism' or naturopathic approaches" (1984:1405). One successful entrepreneur, Michael Harner, resigned his professorship at the New School for Social Research and appears to have developed a lucrative undertaking by offering workshops on shamanic voyages (Hess 1993:150). In early 1994 I detected a pronounced ethos of entrepreneurialism at the San Francisco Whole Life Expo, where chiropractors, Rolfers, health-food proponents, New Agers, psychic healers, and many other alternative practitioners hawked their wares to what appeared to be a predominantly white, middle-class clientele. Goldstein suggests that the holistic health movement may be undergoing a transformation into a "marketed social movement":

> Marketed social movements are characterized by sophisticated promotional and recruitment strategies, a membership that is sharply distinguished from the leadership, participation as a product package, and the growth of membership as a primary goal. . . . Particularly those sectors of the health movement that have been most enmeshed in proprietary organizations rely on professional administrators and exclude most members from decision-making. The social movement becomes a product to be sold to people, regardless of whether they need it. (1992: 151)

The ability of alternative practitioners to attract clients, however, is limited by the fact that many insurance companies do not cover their services. Gordon and Silverstein (1998:91) found that approximately 75 percent of all expenses for alternative health care were paid directly by the patient. Eisenberg et al. (1993, 1998) reported that 64.0 percent of their sample in 1990 and 58.3 percent in 1997 had paid all the costs out-of-pocket for alternative therapy. They estimated that Americans spent $14.6 billion on visits to these practitioners in 1990 and $21.2 billion in 1997.

Perhaps in order to justify to insurers their relatively high costs, alternative practitioners sometimes argue that their treatments will save money in the long run because of their preventive nature. Therapies such as acupuncture, homeopathy, and naturopathy are often labor-intensive and time-consuming, and thus expensive, despite their low-technology orientation. Bratman observes that "individual insurance companies are offering coverage for specific alternative therapies on a case-by-case basis, always making sure to charge more for the coverage than the average costs that will be incurred" (1997:

214). Some insurance companies and HMOs contract alternative practitioners or allow biomedical practitioners to refer patients to them (Gordon and
Silverstein 1998:94). A few insurance companies specialize in plans that cover
alternative therapies. Such companies include Alternative Health Services,
based in Thousand Oaks, California, and American Western Life Insurance
Company, based in Foster City, California.

Because most holistic health services are not covered by insurance policies, Medicare, and Medicaid, their clients tend to be primarily either white,
upper- and upper-middle-class people or members of the counterculture who
have chosen to funnel their often limited financial resources into alternative
health care. The 166 respondents to a questionnaire administered at the San
Andreas Health Council—a holistic health center that houses practitioners
and sponsors classes—tended to have a relatively high socio-economic status
(Mattson 1982:116–22). Their level of education was also high: 7 percent held
doctoral degrees, 19 percent master's degrees, and 39 percent bachelor's degrees; 26 percent had some college education, and only 4 percent had a high
school education or less. In terms of occupation, 35 percent were identified as
being "professional" workers, 17 percent as "helping" workers, 15 percent as
"clerical" workers, 7 percent as "housewives," 8 percent as "students," and 10
percent as "others." Danforth (1989:254) described the typical New Age ad-
herent as a white, upper-middle-class urbanite who grew up during the 1960s
but had been trying to adjust to the more individualistic ethos of the 1980s
and 1990s by seeking emotional intimacy in small groups. Kyle maintains that
"New Agers usually possess a better-than-average education and are urban,
middle class, upwardly mobile, and not particularly alienated from society"
(1995:11). He contends that women constitute about 70 percent of the movement's adherents.

As Salmon observes, the " 'worried well' of middle-age and middle class . . .
has the discretionary income to buy these services from entrepreneurs who
have turned a cosmic ecological concern into a sales package marketed to aid
coping with a stressful social existence" (1984:257). While recognizing that
New Age consciousness contains some positive elements, such as emphasis
on exercise and organic and natural foods, Parenti argues that it exhibits a
form of self-centeredness that "resembles the hyperindividualism of the free-
market society in which it flourishes" and neglects the "common struggle for
collective empowerment and social betterment" (1994:17–18). Danforth contends that one specific New Age healing ritual, firewalking, "generally attracts
people who by most commonly accepted standards would not be considered
'sick' at all" (1989:266). In essence, its adherents are suffering from the general malaise that characterizes much of middle-class life in the United States.

7

Anglo-American Religious and Metaphysical Healing Systems

For historical, social, and cultural reasons, the United States exhibits the greatest degree of religious pluralism of any advanced capitalist society and possibly of any society in the world. Since religion often concerns itself with health matters, it should come as no surprise that many medical systems take on a religious or metaphysical cast. As we have already seen, various heterodox medical systems such as homeopathy, eclecticism, osteopathy, chiropractic, and naturopathy have incorporated metaphysical concepts, although they have often attempted to expunge them as they sought to professionalize themselves. As Horace Miner (1979) so effectively demonstrated in his classic (albeit somewhat tongue-in-cheek) analysis of body ritual among the Nacirema (American spelled roughly backward), even biomedicine exhibits quasi-religious dimensions. He describes the Nacirema as a "magic-ridden" people whose "medicine men" (physicians) perform "elaborate ceremonies" (surgery) in imposing temples, called *latipsos* (hospitals). The medicine men and, increasingly, medicine women are assisted by a "permanent group of vestal maidens [female nurses] who move sedately about the temple chambers in distinctive costume and headdress" (Miner 1979:12).

Because this book attempts to view medical systems as a reflection of hierarchical patterns in American society, and because peoples of Northwestern European ancestry—the so-called WASPs—constitute the dominant ethnic group in the United States, I examine Anglo-American religious healing systems first, in this chapter, before examining those of people of color. In the next chapter I examine the conflation of religion and healing in the folk medical systems of people of color in the United States.

I consider Anglo-American religious and metaphysical healing systems primarily in chronological order. Spiritualism emerged in the 1840s, and various New Thought healing systems, such as Christian Science and Unity, gained ground in the late nineteenth century. Evangelical faith healing also appeared in the late nineteenth century in various Protestant churches, but it took on its most developed form during the early twentieth century within the context of Pentecostalism and later within the neo-Pentecostal, or charismatic, movement. Dianetics and its successor, Scientology, emerged as metaphysical healing systems in the 1950s. In terms of class orientation, Christian Science and Scientology have found their greatest appeal within the upper middle class, and Spiritualism and Unity within the lower middle class. Pentecostalism has attracted mostly working-class and often poor working-class people, whereas the neo-Pentecostal movement has tended to cater to relatively affluent professional people.

SPIRITUALISM AND CHANNELING

Although communication with the spirit realm dates back to the very beginnings of shamanism, it is generally agreed that American Spiritualism per se began with the rappings of the Fox sisters in the 1840s. As is noted in the following chapter, the movement eventually took hold among African Americans, who adapted it to fit their own experience by blending it with other religious and healing traditions. Anglo-American Spiritualism, like Hispanic spiritism, teaches that the disembodied spirit continues to live on after death and that mediums are able to communicate with spirits who can assist mortals in addressing everyday concerns. The *Spiritualist Manual* of the National Spiritualist Association affirms belief in an "Infinite Intelligence" with nature as its expression, and life after death (Ellwood 1973:139).

There are some 450 Spiritualist congregations in the United States. According to Lauer, "although congregations are quite diverse, Spiritualist ministers tend to be similar: middle-aged or older women, with conventional morals, strong wills, and charisma" (1973:488). Unfortunately, little detailed information exists on the social composition of Spiritualist congregations, apart from ethnographic studies conducted by Ellwood (1973), Zaretsky (1974), and Fishman (1979).

Ellwood visited a Spiritualist congregation in a "run-down, inner-city section" of Los Angeles:

> The congregation was mixed; there were blacks, whites, and Mexican-Americans, and young and old, but the leadership was mostly white. All were clearly lower-middle class, dressed in neat, simple clothes. None, not even the young people, showed other than docile external conformity to the norms of respectable, industrious workingmen; there was clearly no long hair or "hip" dress. (1973:137–38)

Zaretsky studied 11 Spiritualist congregations in Bay City (pseudonym), California, which were either affiliated with certain associations, such as the United States Spiritualist Association of Churches and the Universal Spiritual League, or self-incorporated. For the most part, national associations assert relatively little control over their chartered congregations. Zaretsky (1974: 170) describes the social composition of the core members of the congregations he observed as consisting largely of middle-aged singles who had never married or were divorced or widowed, many of whom lived in downtown apartments or residential hotels. Many members were employed as white-collar clerical, secretarial, semi-skilled, or semi-professional workers.

The Unity Science Church studied by Fishman had some 35 members between the ages of 30 and 70. Over half of the members were widows or housewives over age 60; 90 percent of the members were white and 10 percent were African American. Although the congregation was situated in a lower-to lower-middle-class blue-collar neighborhood, most of its members did not reside close to the church.

Spiritualism is a religious movement that views ritual and health as intricately intertwined. Spiritualists believe that some diseases are caused by spirit possession (Fishman 1979:10) and others by the "seed of thought" embedded in a person's mind. Healers assert that "at least some spirits, called *guides,* are concerned for the health of living persons and willing to provide their healing services via a medium" (Lee 1976:31). The Spiritualist healer seeks to "direct astral energy (often by the movement of the hands, as well as by positive thought), under the guidance of the healing spirit" (Lee 1976:32). Healers may specialize in curing certain diseases, depending upon the spirit guide's reputation when he or she was alive. Some Spiritualist healers claimed that a "healing odic force" (a term derived from Odin, the ancient Norse god) flows from their fingers (Judah 1967:70). Others claim that they can discover the source of disease by examining the client's aura.

Spiritualist churches in Bay City offered two forms of public service to their members and clients: messages presented in response to a client's question about personal problems or in the form of a sermon addressed to the entire congregation, and the laying on of hands for those who sought help for physical ailments or mental disorders. Messages came from the spirits or from God, who was referred to as Infinite Intelligence. Spiritualist pastors and mediums in Bay City also conducted private readings for their clients:

> This is regarded by most Spiritualists as the most desirable form of communication with the spirits because the medium can speak privately and therefore does not have to shield what the spirits say. . . . When an individual comes to a private reading, he [or she] usually chats with the medium for a few moments in order to warm the atmosphere. Then the medium will ask the client whether he [or she] would prefer to talk or be talked to. . . . It is expected that the medium will bring forth from the spirit some information which will pertain to the need, question, or worry of the client. As the information is produced, the client indicates some kind of recognition of whether the information is accurate or whether there is need for further talk by the medium in order to hit the point at issue. Once the

problem has been mentioned, the medium will converse with the client about it. (Zaretsky 1974:206)

The Unity Science Church in Buffalo provided three healing methods: prayer healing, which occurred during a healing service; faith healing, which was performed by a spiritual healer; and magnetic healing, or laying on of hands, which occurred during private healing ceremonies for serious illnesses (Fishman 1979:12–15). Following the service, a healing ceremony took place in a private healing chamber. Clients chose the healer whom they wanted to treat them. While the client was seated, a group of church members stood in a circle around the client and healer. The healer invoked the "Christ Principle of Healing," then placed her or his hands on the client's neck or head, and psychically determined the ailment and bodily area that needed treatment. As the healer touched, massaged, or manipulated the afflicted area, the church members offered healing energy through prayer. According to Fishman, "in those cases in which healing fails to take place, the church believes that the individual was not a believer and that the patient is not fulfilling his obligations to the principles set forth within this church" (1979:16).

The movement that is in many ways the successor to Spiritualism, which has gone into a period of decline since its zenith in the nineteenth century, is channeling—a phenomenon that is part of the New Age movement discussed in the previous chapter. Anthropologist Michael F. Brown maintains that "channeling incorporates features of nineteenth-century American spiritualism, including the recovery movement and women-centered spirituality" (1997:6), but channeling adherents generally do not recognize the historical link with Spiritualism. Its practitioners claim that they can establish contact with spiritual guides from earlier historical eras and mythological places. J. Z. Knight, a renowned channel, believes that her body serves as a vessel for Ramtha, the Enlightened One, an Atlantean warrior and deity. Ramtha asserts that earthquakes, volcanic eruptions, floods, and climatic changes will propel humans into a New Age in which they will be able to realize their true potential as gods. Channels conduct workshops throughout the country that teach adherents how to contact their spiritual guides and guardian angels. There are two types of channels: trance channels, who claim to undergo a complete separation from their bodies while channeling, and conscious channels, who remain aware of their surroundings while channeling. Channeling adherents tend to believe that "God resides within each of us" and that reincarnation occurs (Babbie 1990:261).

Brown presents the following socioeconomic profile of channels and their clients:

People involved specifically in channeling fit the general profile of Boomers who find their way into other NRMs [New Religious Movements]. There is, however,

124

a significant demographic split between the producers and consumers of chan-
neled information. The consumers—those who attend channeling workshops or
seek individual counseling—are well educated and often affluent. Channels—
the producers in this exchange—have educational backgrounds similar to their
clients, but their economic situation is often precarious because of their unusual
career. Some channels use channeling as their primary means of income. Others
have ordinary jobs and try to fit channeling activities into their free time. The
professional channels who enjoy the most stable incomes are those who manage
to integrate channeling into a conventional occupation, often as psychotherapists
or motivational trainers. (1997:7–8)

While most channels have to supplement the income they derive from
channeling, a few channels have developed lucrative practices. Jach Pusel, a
former insurance agent from Michigan who serves as a channel for Lazaris,
operates Concept:Synergy, a company that employs "a dozen people and gen-
erates millions of dollars annually, through sales of *The Lazaris Materials*:
videos (up to $59.95 each), sets of audiocasettes (up to $24.95), and books (as
much as $12.95 each)" (D'Antonio 1992:112).

As was also true in the Spiritualist movement, women tend to be more involved in channeling, both as channels and as clients, than men, sometimes
by a ratio of 3:1 or greater (Brown 1997:95). Female channels do not generally identify with the feminist movement, however, and often have male spirit
guides. Channeling adherents have by and large eschewed the establishment
of religious congregations. They tend to see themselves as embarked upon a
quest for "spirituality" rather an effort to establish hierarchical religious organizations per se. As Brown observes, "today's channels share with yesterday's
spiritualists the belief that American freedoms include the right, perhaps even
the duty, to pursue growth beyond the arbitrary limits set by institutions"
(1997:118). Fellowship tends to occur within the context of informal self-help
groups and professional counseling sessions or group workshops. Nevertheless, a few channeling congregations have been established. The Temple of
Light Ascendant—one of the two congregations visited by Michael Brown—
maintains an informal affiliation with the National Spiritualist Association of
Churches (Brown 1997:135).

While Spiritualism and channeling exhibit some striking similarities, the
former has done much more to develop a congregational life than has the
latter, at least thus far. Macklin (1974:383) maintains that Spiritualism constitutes a ritual "drama of salvation" that seeks to heal the split between the
temporal and spiritual orders, and Fishman (1979:17) asserts that Spiritualism serves to reincorporate its adherents into the larger society. In essence,
Spiritualism provides many individuals who are socially isolated with a sense
of community, although often a rather transitory one. Although Spiritualist
congregations have some core members, both Spiritualism and channeling

function largely as "client cults" (Stark and Bainbridge 1985:208–33), or what I prefer to refer to as "client sects." Client sects tend to propagate their doctrines primarily by way of dyadic relationships between a therapist (or consultant) and a client (or patient). In the case of Spiritualist congregations in Bay City, "about 70 percent of the congregation changes from week to week, and one continuously faces a group of persons who either attend the church infrequently or are newcomers" (Zaretsky 1974:216).

Both Spiritualist mediums and New Age channels tend to focus on private concerns. According to Fishman, Spiritualism serves to "alleviate the emotional responses that are an inherent part of most illness situations" (1979: 20). Channels generally maintain that people's current problems result from fears or unresolved conflicts that occurred in an earlier life. They assert that people create their own reality and tend to downplay or deny social factors that may contribute to misfortune or illness. Like many proponents of positive thinking, certain channels teach that affluent people have attained financial prosperity because of their positive attitude and that the poor live with scarcity because they are too negative. Despite their metaphysical overtones, both Spiritualist mediums and New Age channels take an approach similar to that of conventional psychotherapists, who often urge their clients to muster the psychic resources necessary to adjust to the demands of the larger society. Whereas nineteenth-century Spiritualism supported various types of social reforms, twentieth-century Spiritualism has evolved into a highly introversionist and individualistic effort. Many channeling adherents maintain that they are sowing the seeds for the development of a global community; however, they fail to answer the "question of how the new global village will build schools, repair streets, collect garbage, and keep the peace" (Brown 1997: 125). Even while espousing a more egalitarian and democratic social order, channels tend to focus on private concerns and thus reinforce strongly ingrained patterns of individualism in American society.

In essence, both Spiritualism and channeling contribute to the "cult of private life" championed by such agencies of socialization as the family, the schools, the mass media, advertising, and social workers, and which serves to legitimize the existing social system. As Greisman and Mayers so astutely observe, according to this perspective, "the source, if not the cause, of mental disorders is invariably traced to the client himself and/or his friends and relations" (1977:61).

NEW THOUGHT RELIGIOUS HEALING SYSTEMS

New Thought "began as a late nineteenth-century New England healing movement within self-consciously Christian circles" (Alexander 1992:35). It

126

emerged in New England as a blend of the notions of "manifest destiny" and "progress"; a "Horatio Alger–type optimism about the possibilities of self-improvement" through positive thinking and affirmation; and Transcendentalism, a philosophical orientation based upon the ideas of figures such as Emerson and Thoreau, who emphasized the transcendence of industrial civilization by retreating into the inner soul and nature (Lee 1976:28). Later it spread to other parts of the country, particularly the Midwest and the West Coast. In New Thought, God is the omnipotent and omnipresent source of power and energy and a force that resides in all individuals. Adherents of New Thought groups maintain that the mind can solve all human problems; they rely upon mind cure, mental cure, or metaphysical healing, and believe that affirmation—the process of "affirming the state of being one wishes to have"—can assist an individual in attaining "happiness, peace of mind, prosperity, etc., in addition to health" (Judah 1967:187).

Although Christian Scientists have resisted them, efforts have been made to bring adherents of various New Thought groups together under a common organizational umbrella. These have included the Divine Science Association (est. 1892), the International Metaphysical League, and the New Thought Alliance (Meyer 1965:36–37). The New Thought Alliance consisted of Unity centers, the Divine and Religious Science congregations, and Churches of the Higher Life.

CHRISTIAN SCIENCE

Christian Science constitutes the most organized manifestation of the New Thought movement (Gottschalk 1973). It denies the existence of matter, sin, death, and sickness, and asserts that all is mind (Christian Science Publishing Society 1990). It is a religious healing system that claims to eradicate all manner of disease through spiritual power. Singer (1982:3) delineates six stages in the structural evolution of Christian Science: (1) the germinal phase (1866–1872), during which Mary Baker Eddy developed her ideas about healing; (2) the cultic phase (1873–1880), during which a loosely organized group assembled around Eddy; (3) the sectarian phase (1891–1890), entailing growth, diffusion, and bureaucratization; (4) the transitional phase (1891–1930), following the death of Eddy, when leadership became concentrated in a board of directors; (5) the institutional phase (1931–1970), entailing completion of a formal bureaucratic structure and rising status of its membership; and (6) a decline, characterized by decreasing membership, at least in the United States, and internal conflict.

The Church of Christ, Scientist, has an elaborate centralized bureaucracy with ultimate authority vested in the Mother Church in Boston, which prepares weekly texts based on *Science and Health* that are used in religious services and reading rooms. Christian Science does not have a clergy per se, but has its own professional body of teachers and health practitioners. The board of directors has complete authority over the governing and doctrinal content of the Church. Although branch churches elect their own officers, all officers are accountable to the central board. By 1900, the organization claimed to encompass nearly 500 congregations in North America and Europe. Since then, it has grown to some 3,000 branches in 50 countries (Gottschalk 1990:11). It is difficult to determine membership figures, since the church does not publicize them. Estimates indicate that membership may have reached 400,000 during the 1960s, but recent reports suggest a decline in the United States, Britain, and elsewhere (Simmons 1995:66). The Christian Science church publishes the *Christian Science Monitor,* a well-respected, general newspaper read by many non-Scientists.

The Christian Science Sunday morning service dispenses with the conventional Protestant minister and emphasizes gender equality by having the ritual led by two congregationally elected readers, who are always a woman and a man. The lay readers read aloud from *Science and Health.* At a service in the "Extension" or "Annex" of the Mother Church, which was completed in 1904 and houses 5,000 people, Gill observed "at most 400" attendees (1998:xii). More than half of the hour-long service consisted of pairs of quotations, with a woman reading from the Bible and then a man reading from *Science and Health with Key to the Scriptures.* The sedate service also included hymns in which Christian Science words were set to some traditional Protestant tunes. Gill saw about 200 people attending the Sunday evening service in the Mother Church (1998:xii). Church Science congregations generally conduct testimonial meetings on Wednesday evenings at which members speak about personal healing experiences. Christian Scientists tend to be upper-middle-class, well-educated, professional people, and are predominantly women. As Bloom so aptly observes, "urban and rural masses do not become Christian Scientists. To deny the reality of matter and of the body you must be very clean, well fed and housed and clothed, and easily able to afford medical care when benign animal magnetism falls short" (1992:145).

Despite its aura of respectability, Christian Science has not escaped the animosity of organized biomedicine. In the 1890s, for example, "the AMA . . . had launched all-out war against Christian Science" (Peel 1988:111). According to Weitz,

> Christian Scientists' opposition to medical care has precipitated a long history of legal battles in which doctors or the state have sued for the right to force individuals to accept medical treatment. In general, courts have ruled that because Christian Scientists never seek medical care, doctors have no legal standing and cannot force care on adults. However, courts have ruled in favor of forcing care

on children, arguing that the state has the right and duty to protect the health of children. (1996:291)

Indeed, in 1988 and 1989, four sets of Christian Science parents were convicted for manslaughter or neglect in the deaths of their children for refusing to seek biomedical care for them (Cockerham 1995:139). For the most part, however, Christian Science and biomedicine have reached a rapprochement of sorts. Christian Scientists generally resort to biomedical treatment as a stop-gap method until they have more fully developed their mental power over disease. Conversely, particularly in recent years, biomedicine has been forced, largely due to external pressure, to more fully appreciate the interaction of physiological and emotional processes.

Historians and journalists have given more attention to Christian Science than have sociologists and anthropologists. In contrast to the former, who have tended to focus on the life of Mary Baker Eddy and the organizational development of the church that she established, the latter have been interested in Christian Science as a religious healing system. Christian Science treatment strives to be entirely and exclusively metaphysical. Fox (1989:109) maintains that despite its attempt to avoid psychological processes, Christian Science relies upon a psychosomatic theory of disease. As Wilson observes, Christian Scientists view prayer as "neither praise nor supplication, but an attempt to bring subjective attitudes in accord with what Science proclaims to be objective reality" (1966:43–44).

Although any Christian Scientist is in theory competent to heal himself or herself, a practitioner's assistance is thought to facilitate the process. Christian Science practitioners receive a Bachelor of Christian Science following completion of a two-week course. Practitioners are self-recruited through several different routes (Fox 1989:103). The January 1985 issue of the *Journal* enumerated 2,884 practitioners, 725 of whom practiced in California, 82 in Washington State, and 63 in Oregon (Schoepflin 1988:212). Given that its founder was a woman, it is not surprising that women have played a prominent role as healers in Christian Science. According to Schoepflin (1988:199), the female:male ratio for practitioners was 5:1 in the 1890s and had risen to 8:1 by the early 1970s. Wardwell (1965:180) reported that women constituted 77 percent of all full-time practitioners in 1953. Women also overwhelmingly predominate in the role of Christian Science nurse—a status which Eddy approved in 1908. The 1985 *Christian Science Journal* listed 480 certified nurses in the United States, whose responsibilities entail caring for patients and assisting practitioners by holding pure thoughts that make a positive contribution to the healing atmosphere. Whereas women predominate in therapeutic positions, men predominate in the more prestigious, higher-paying administrative and teaching positions (Fox 1989:100). Several states allow

Christian Science practitioners to sign sick leave certificates and disability claims (Weiss and Lonnquist 1997:232). Christian Science practitioners and nurses receive coverage under Medicare, Medicaid, government employee insurance plans, many health insurance companies, and Blue Cross/Blue Shield in several states. The Internal Revenue Service recognizes practitioners' fees as "medical expenses" that may be deductible for those who itemize deductions.

Christian Science healing relies upon prayer, mental work, and Eddy's *Science and Health with Key to the Scriptures* and is founded upon the belief that reading and praying lead to acquisition of the spark of the divine mind that Jesus possessed. The Christian Science practitioner helps her or his client to recognize that health is natural and that sin, sickness, and death are not real. Singer (1982:4) maintains that practitioners focus more on the treatment of particular ailments than on determining their cause.

Christian Science is essentially this-worldly and seeks to promote the worldly success of its adherents. It tends to embrace a liberal humanitarianism by emphasizing a relatively active social ethic of aiding and treating such global problems as natural disasters, political conflict, and social crises (Schoepflin 1988:213). In contrast, its acceptance of class and gender hierarchies makes it a hegemonic institution. The Christian Science church provides women with an alternative vehicle for status recognition in the roles of practitioner and nurse without at the same time challenging the basic gender hierarchy of the larger society.

Based upon his research on Christian Science healing and alcoholism psychotherapy, Singer (1982:10) concludes that Christian Science reflects the "core values of Western society—values that often disguise the structural realities" of advanced capitalist societies such as the United States. It teaches that the individual can completely overcome her or his urge to drink by recognizing that alcohol lacks power to control the human mind. The Christian Science approach to alcoholism is similar to that of conventional psychotherapy —both "express a shared assumption: alcoholism is an individual problem rather than a reflection of more general structural contradictions in the larger society" (Singer 1982:8). This observation confirms DeHood's assertion that Christian Science constitutes "an opiate for those whose lives are already sheltered" (1937:175).

Like other successful religious movements, Christian Science spawned a number of splinter groups. Emma Curtis Hopkins, a disciple of Mary Baker Eddy, separated herself from her mentor in 1885 and indirectly contributed to the emergence of a number of rival New Thought bodies. She moved to Chicago in 1885 and established in 1886 what became known as the Christian Science Theological Seminary. According to Melton,

During the decade from 1886 through 1895, Hopkins trained a number of students who went on to found these "denominations" which today constitute the core of the New Thought tradition. Among her students were Melinda Cramer (founder of Divine Science), Myrtle and Charles Fillmore (founders of the Unity School of Christianity), Annie Rix Militz (founder of the Homes of Truth), and Kate Bingham (who in turned trained Nona Brooks, who founded Divine Science in Denver, Colorado). In the years after leaving Chicago and settling in New York City Hopkins taught Clara Stocker (who in turn would teach Albert Grier, the founder of the Church of Truth) and Ernest Holmes (who founded Religious Science). (1992:16–17)

UNITY SCHOOL OF CHRISTIANITY

Next to Christian Science, the Unity School of Christianity is the largest New Thought group. Myrtle Fillmore (1845–1931) and Charles Fillmore (1854–1948) took a series of courses with Eugene B. Weeks, a Christian Science practitioner, in the spring of 1886 and also a class with Joseph Adams, another Christian Science practitioner, in the summer of 1887 in Kansas City, Missouri (Vahle 1996:208–12). Myrtle's contact with Christian Science reportedly cured her of tuberculosis. She became a Christian Science practitioner in 1887 and also studied with Emma Curtis Hopkins initially in Kansas City and later in Chicago. Hopkins ordained Myrtle Fillmore on December 15, 1890. Charles Fillmore, a real-estate agent in Kansas City, Missouri, lost $150,000 in a recession that struck the Midwest (D'Andrade 1974:20, 28). He became impressed when his wife's spiritual endeavors resulted in healing. Through prayer and meditation, Charles himself obtained relief from a dislocated hip and a leg condition that required him to wear a brace to support his right leg, which was some three inches shorter than his left leg.

In April 1889 the Fillmores abandoned their secular occupations and started publishing a periodical entitled *Modern Thought*. They established a prayer ministry the following year. The Fillmores attempted to create a "practical" Christianity aimed at people of all denominations. They regarded Unity more as a "school" than a church per se. Over the course of their involvement with Unity, Myrtle functioned primarily as a healer whereas Charles functioned more as an administrator and the author of numerous religious books. The theological underpinnings of Unity, however, evolved as a collaborative effort of the Fillmores as well as other Unity practitioners.

In addition to Christian Science, the Fillmores were influenced by Swedenborgianism, Transcendentalism, Spiritualism, Theosophy, Hinduism, and Rosicrucianism. Like other New Thought and metaphysical groups, Unity views Jesus Christ as an exemplary figure rather than as a messiah who will deliver humanity from its sins. It views each person as the individualized expression of the Divine Mind, maintains that individuals have total control of their lives, and emphasizes meditation as a means of getting in touch with one's inner self. Heaven and hell are seen as states of mind rather than specific places where a person goes following death. Myrtle Fillmore taught that the "mind could be made to focus on the thoughts and ideas that produced health rather than illness, plenty rather than poverty, and satisfying human relationships rather than unhappy ones" (Vahle 1996:6). She maintained that "right thinking" could solve an individual physical, psychological, or spiritual problem as well as social problems. Disease originated in thoughts held in the mind. Myrtle held a low opinion of prescription drugs, advocated vegetarianism and abstinence from red meat, asserted that "human beings could—through the proper understanding and application of Truth Principles—regenerate the cells of their bodies, remain youthful and vigorous despite advancing years, and ultimately overcome physical death, and taught a form of reincarnation" (Vahle 1996:92).

The Fillmores began to purchase land outside of Kansas City in 1920 and established the headquarters of their "school" at Unity Village in Lee's Summit, Missouri. Unity broke its affiliation with the New Thought Alliance in 1906, rejoined it in 1919, and disaffiliated itself again in 1922 (Meyer 1965:41). In 1992 it reportedly had 602 congregations and 166 study groups (deChant 1993:102). Unity operates a 24-hour pray ministry called "Silent Unity" which responds to some 2 million prayer requests each year, the largest religious publishing house in the Midwest, a school of religious education at Unity Village with an annual enrollment of some 1,500 students, and a seminary (Vahle 1996:xi). The *Daily Word,* an inspirational publication, has a circulation of 1.2 million and is distributed in 153 countries.

Unity allows its members to belong to other religious bodies. Each Unity center operates independently and may take on distinct characteristics. In her brief ethnographic overview of two Unity congregations, McGuire (1991:23) observed that the smaller center, identified as the "Unity Church of Christ," was warmer and more oriented toward traditional Christianity, exemplified by the prominent display of a large portrait of Jesus on the wall behind the podium. In contrast, the larger center was eclectic in its belief system and tended to emphasize more individualistic concerns. In addition to seeking inner tranquility and wellness, some Unity congregations emphasize the acquisition of financial prosperity through positive thinking and rituals of affirmation.

Unity views health as the achievement of oneness with the Christ Mind. Illness results from disharmony in mind and body and occurs only when people permit it to enter their consciousness. Healing is a "mind process" in that it entails altering one's modes of thought and speech and can be directed to a broad

132

range of economic, political, and social issues. Unity deemphasizes diagnostic approaches but stresses four therapeutic techniques: affirmation or the statement of a desired, positive condition; denial and release of negative thoughts; relaxation exercises; and meditation. Healing is believed to occur through scrupulous study of Unity's many publications. A Unity handbook asserts that numerous diseases including syphilis, can be cured by "profound realization of truth" and that epidemics can by eradicated by "quietly, confidently, peacefully knowing" their non-existence (quoted in Lee 1976:32–33). Charles Fillmore articulated the Unity philosophy of healing in *Christian Healing* (1909) and *Jesus Christ Heals* (1939). Historically, Unity has had a much more harmonious relationship with biomedicine than has Christian Science. Adherents of Unity freely utilize biomedicine and other medical systems. However, McGuire (1982:89) reported that her Unity informants in suburban New Jersey maintained that authentic healing had to take place within the person.

In keeping with Unity's eclectic predilections, many of its congregations have drawn upon New Age beliefs and practices. Indeed, as Melton observes,

> As the New Age movement grew in prominence, the boundaries between New Thought and New Age became increasingly blurred. At this point, a reaction began to take place as New Thought leaders took a critical look at the movement's agenda. Unity minister Dell de Chant has noted a growing resistance in New Thought to what became increasingly seen as New Age encroachment. . . .
> . . . The Unity of Christianity, whose president, Connie Fillmore, had become concerned about New Age distortions of Unity teachings, removed New Age material from its center in Unity Village, Missouri. Though the leaders of the Association of Unity Churches share Fillmore's anti–New Age bias, they had less luck in removing *A Course in the Miracles* classes from the independent-minded local churches and the New Age paraphernalia from the bookrooms. (1992:27)

Like Christian Science and other metaphysical groups, Unity tends to assume a relatively apolitical stance on social issues. Although Myrtle Fillmore was a Republican who exemplified a prototypical midwestern conservatism, she did not advise her followers how to vote. She believed that Unity should help people to evolve spiritually at an individual level rather than to solve social problems. Myrtle maintained that the Great Depression was a byproduct of negative thinking rather than of Herbert Hoover's economic policies and that Unity's mission was not "to make homes for the homeless or to take in those who need special care and rest" (quoted in Vahle 1996:37). In his book *Prosperity* (1936), Charles Fillmore emphasized spiritual substance over money but asserted that financial prosperity comes out of the former (D'Andrade 1974:94). Many Unity adherents view wealth or affluence as a significant byproduct of spiritual development.

SPIRITUAL FRONTIERS FELLOWSHIP

In contrast to Christian Science and Unity, the Spiritual Frontiers Fellowship (SFF) is a relatively recent New Thought organization. SFF was established in 1956 in Evanston, Illinois, by 75 religious leaders and laypersons and achieved a membership of almost 8,000 by 1975. The organization's primary concerns are prayer, healing, and immortality. Anthropologist Melinda Bollar Wagner (1983) conducted fieldwork on the Metro Area study group (situated in a midwestern urban area) affiliated with SFF. Metro Area meetings were held every month, were attended by some 50 to 75 people, and consisted of a healing service, a short meditation, a lecture, and a "coffee hour." SFF's smaller, local study groups met more frequently and consisted of only eight to twelve members. Study groups devoted a considerable amount of attention to members' personal problems. SFF teaches that each person must find his or her own path to truth. Like members of other metaphysical groups, SFF adherents seek self-realization and a happier adjustment to everyday life. Study group members tend to form warm and intimate but often transitory relations with one another (Wagner 1983:163). Wagner asserts that SFF and other metaphysical groups address a sense of alienation that many Americans face in an increasingly socially fragmented society. SFF embodies the American core values of individualism and pragmatism and appeals to "middle Americans" seeking to improve their socio-economic status.

EVANGELICAL FAITH HEALING, PENTECOSTALISM, AND THE CHARISMATIC MOVEMENT

Protestant reformers rejected many of the healing rituals and beliefs in healing miracles that had long been associated with Roman Catholicism. In the late nineteenth century, however, Evangelical Protestants began to develop an interest in faith healing. Faith healers take their inspiration from biblical descriptions of healings performed by Jesus. The most explicit biblical passage comes from James 5:14–16:

> Is any sick among you? Let him call for the elders of the church; and let them pray over him, anointing him with oil in the name of the Lord: And the prayer of faith shall save the sick man and the Lord shall raise him up; if he have committed sins, they shall be forgiven him.

The first "faith cure" convention occurred in Philadelphia in June 1882 (Cunningham 1974:504). John Alexander Dowie, a Congregational minister, was the first widely known healing evangelist in the United States (Harrell 1988:217). In 1900 he purchased 6,000 acres midway between Chicago and

134

Milwaukee where he built Zion City, which eventually boasted a population of over 10,000. Dowie relied heavily on healing to attract followers, and he condemned physicians and regular medicine. Although he rejected speaking in tongues, or glossolalia, he became a role model for a future generation of Pentecostal evangelists who practiced divine healing (Harrell 1988:221). The heyday of the faith healing revival occurred in the two decades following World War II (Harrell 1988). The revival contained two wings: a moderate group represented by Oral Roberts, who promoted a merger of biomedicine and divine healing, and a radical group led by A. A. Allen and Jack Coe, who denounced biomedicine and physicians.

ANGLO-AMERICAN PENTECOSTALISM

Over the course of the twentieth century, faith healing manifested itself most explicitly within the Pentecostal movement. To a large extent, this movement constituted a radical extension of the Holiness movement that had developed in various mainstream denominations following the Civil War. Harrell (1975: 11) identified several sites where the Pentecostal movement emerged: a center in western North Carolina and eastern Tennessee connected with A. J. Tomlinson and the Church of God; a center in Topeka, Kansas, associated with Reverend Charles Parham, who left his congregation in order to practice faith healing and speaking in tongues; and the interracial Azusa Street revival of 1906–1909 in Los Angeles.

Parham left the Methodist Episcopal Church to form Bethel Healing Home in Topeka in 1898 (Synan 1971:100). He had been inspired by the healing ministry of J. A. Dowie of Zion City and visited Holiness and healing ministries from Chicago to New York to Georgia in 1900. In the fall of 1900, Parham established the Bethel Bible College in Topeka. Some of his students began to speak in tongues in early 1901 after investigating the doctrine of the "baptism of the Spirit." Parham closed his college and instructed his students to spread the message of the new Pentecost. He opened another Bible college in Houston in 1905 and recruited William Seymour, an African American Holiness preacher affiliated with the Church of God in Anderson, Indiana. Seymour in turn served as the inspiration for the famous revival at the Azusa Street Mission in Los Angeles. Because of Seymour's role in the revival, Tinney contends that he was the "father of modern-day Pentecostalism," despite being overlooked "by those who are contemptible of his race" (1978:213). In addition to an interracial audience drawn from the "poorest of the lower classes" (Synan 1971:107), many prospective converts and curiosity seekers from all over the United States as well as many other countries attended the revival. Some of the "third blessed" returned home to establish Pentecostal groups of their own. G. B. Cashwell, a white Holiness preacher from North Carolina, repressed his racial prejudice and asked Seymour and several of his black assistants to lay hands on his head so that he could be filled with the Holy Ghost. After receiving the Spirit, he spread the Pentecostal gospel to many people, both white and black, in the Southeast. In early 1907, Charles H. Mason, J. A. Peter, and D. J. Young also spoke in tongues during their five-week stay at the Azusa Street Mission. After he returned to his headquarters in Memphis, Mason asked an assembly of the Church of God in Christ to transform the sect into a Pentecostal group—a move that forced his compatriot C. P. Jones to form the Church of Christ (Holiness) U.S.A. (Cobbins 1966).

The initial interracial character of the Pentecostal movement began to break down in the years following the Asuza Street revival. Both before and after 1906, C. H. Mason ordained many white ministers of independent congregations because the Church of God in Christ was one of the few legally incorporated Holiness-Pentecostal bodies in the mid-South. According to Anderson, "the whites appear to have operated independently, using the name Church of God in Christ (COGIC) with no indication of its connection with the black group, and publishing their own official organ, Word and Witness" (1979:213). In 1914, COGIC-ordained white ministers formed the Assemblies of God in Hot Springs, Arkansas. The division along racial lines of the Pentecostal Assemblies of the World, which initially had "roughly equal numbers of Negroes and whites as both officials and members," formally ended the interracial period in American Pentecostalism in 1924 (Synan 1971:221).

Pentecostalism initially made its strongest appeal to both white and black working-class and lower-class people (Quebedeaux 1983:3–4; Synan 1997: 203). In his biographical analysis of 45 early Pentecostal leaders (only two of whom were black), Anderson observed that the prototypical Pentecostal leader was a "comparatively young man of humble rural-agrarian origins" who was often a "victim of physical as well as cultural and economic deprivation" but who "managed to secure a smattering of advanced education of relatively low quality" (1979:113). He also noted that the Pentecostal movement drew the "overwhelming bulk of its recruits from the working poor," most of whom were semi-skilled and unskilled laborers (Anderson 1979:223). Pentecostalism substituted high religious status for its adherents' low social status:

> Pentecostalism is often seen as a form of popular religion and therefore has very little prestige in the eyes of the wider society. Pentecostals themselves feel a certain pride and even superiority toward the rest of society. Experiences with healing and other charismatic gifts nourish this feeling of superiority. Real human destiny, they feel, does not depend on society's notions and views. This attitude is only possible because the personal relation with God gives the believers the certainty of being on the right track. Religious power, nourished by the experience of wholeness, is the basis for social behavior. (Droogers 1994:47–48)

Although the Pentecostal movement found its greatest appeal in the South, it spread to other parts of the country often as a result of southerners' migrating to the Midwest and the West in search of better economic opportunities. Anderson (1979:223) regarded the Pentecostal movement as "one small part of a widespread, long-term protest against modern urban-industrial capitalist society" and modernity. Despite its populist origins, white Pentecostalism quickly developed into a largely reactionary and racist movement that deflected attention away from the political-economic roots of its adherents' plight. Pentecostalists refused to join labor unions, political parties, fraternal lodges, and other organizations (Anderson 1979:229).

Anglo-American Pentecostalism (like African American Pentecostalism) has a rich history of colorful and even flamboyant evangelists. Aimee Semple McPherson, a former Assemblies of God minister who went on to establish the International Church of the Foursquare Gospel, took the country by storm during the 1920s with her evangelical message and faith healing. In the 1940s, Oral Roberts created a "faith-healing empire" and radio (and later, television) ministry based in Tulsa (Synan 1997:215). In 1965, along with R. O. Corvin, he established Oral Roberts University in Tulsa, which later included a medical center. In 1968, Roberts, who had been a Pentecostal Holiness Church evangelist, took a step toward middle-class respectability by affiliating himself with the Methodist church. Pentecostal healers such as Oral Roberts and Katherine Kuhlman often functioned as "bridges to a non-Pentecostal audience who sought healings at their hands" (Poloma 1982:86). Old-line members of the Pentecostal movement came to refer to converts from mainstream churches as "neo-Pentecostals" (Synan 1997:215).

Following World War II, more and more Pentecostalists had either achieved modest levels of affluence or were recruited from the ranks of the lower-middle and even upper-middle classes. Sociologist Margaret Poloma found that, in a sample of 1,275 Assemblies of God adherents, 22 percent were college graduates and only 17 percent had not graduated from high school (Poloma 1989:6). She also reported that 47 percent of her respondents had annual incomes over $15,000 and observed that the Assemblies of God had evolved into a respectable religious body based largely in suburban areas (Poloma 1989:17).

Pentecostalists have historically regarded healing as one of the nine gifts of the Holy Spirit. Indeed, Anderson (1979:93) contends that healing was a significant "drawing card" for the Pentecostal movement. Although Aimee Semple McPherson brought faith healing to public attention through radio broadcasts, healing became commonplace within the Pentecostal movement as a result of the ministries of evangelists such as William M. Branham, A. A. Allen, and Oral Roberts. According to Williams,

> Cancer . . . was one of the most popular matters for curing. Many others were cured as well, and the extraordinary A. A. Allen claimed to have healed, among other things, a case of hermaphroditism. Many of the more extreme evangelists stressed their role as exorcists, and performed their cures through the casting out of the demons allegedly responsible for both mental and physical illness. . . . Even more spectacularly, these healers resurrected occasional clients from the dead. (1980:148)

Faith or divine healing relies upon praying, laying on of hands, anointing with holy oil, and use of prayer cloths and aprons. Riscalla (1975:168) views healings resulting from the laying on of hands as a result of the placebo effect or the power of suggestion.

Anderson (1979:236–39), whose analysis remains the most insightful one to date, argues that Anglo-American Pentecostalism serves several functions, none of which seriously challenges the larger society or significantly alters the position of Pentecostals within in it. Pentecostalism, he contends, (1) constitutes a cathartic mechanism for marginalized people; (2) provides career opportunities for its leaders; (3) serves as a "safety valve" for dissatisfaction within mainstream churches; (4) facilitates the migration process from the countryside to the city; (5) instills in its members passivity, industriousness, and thrift; and (6) develops a compliant working class.

THE CHARISMATIC MOVEMENT

While Pentecostalism proper has catered largely to lower-middle- or working-class people, neo-Pentecostalism, or the charismatic movement, has tended on the whole to cater to more affluent people, ranging from those of lower-middle-class to upper-middle-class status (Quebedeaux 1983:11). As Harrell observed, neo-Pentecostalism "ministers to a joyfully upwardly mobile middle class" and constitutes a "culture-affirming, success-oriented movement which sells its wares in glittering buildings and on slickly produced television programs" (1988:225). Indeed, the charismatic movement first spread among some members of mainstream Protestant churches (e.g. Episcopalians, Lutherans, and Presbyterians) in the 1950s and among Roman Catholics in the 1960s (McGuire 1982:4; Csordas 1994:16).

In addition to Oral Roberts, two individuals in particular promoted the Protestant wing of the neo-Pentecostal or charismatic movement. Demos Shakarian established the Full Gospel Business Men in 1952 and David du Plessis, a South African-born Assemblies of God pastor in Connecticut, established connections with mainstream churches by joining the World Council of Churches in 1954 and attending the Vatican II conference as the sole Pentecostal observer. Despite being excommunicated from the Assemblies of God in 1962, du Plessis went on to become a catalyst in sparking the charismatic movement in mainstream churches (Synan 1997:221). The charismatic movement also received an infusion of energy in the form of the "Jesus People revolution," a youth revival that began in California but quickly spread to other parts of the country. Pat Robertson, Jim Bakker, and Jimmy Swaggart joined Oral Roberts as highly visible and influential charismatic televangelists.

Sociologist Margaret Poloma (1982:87–92) identified three primary forms of healing among Protestant charismatics: healing through private prayer, healing through congregational prayer, and special healing services. Whereas traditional Pentecostalists tend to eschew visualization because they fear that the devil may intrude into this ritual, McGuire (1982:223) reported that her Protestant charismatic (as well as Catholic charismatic) subjects in suburban New Jersey believed that visualization of a past traumatic event could function as a means of confronting its associated pain. In contrast to the hostility between many early Pentecostalists and biomedical physicians, contemporary charismatics teach that physicians are instruments for divine healing. Conversely, many physicians and nurses have come to seek the merits of "touch therapy," including laying on of hands.

The Pentecostal movement within Catholicism began in the spring of 1967 at Duquesne University in Pittsburgh, but then spread to Notre Dame University and to students at Michigan State University. Members of the Catholic Pentecostal movement initially referred to themselves as "pentecostal Catholics" or "Catholic pentecostals," but later designated themselves as "Catholic charismatics" for class reasons (McGuire 1982:4).

Although journalists and historians have given considerable attention to Protestant charismatics, particularly those affiliated with the religious Right, the most in-depth social scientific studies of the charismatic movement have focused on Catholic charismatics (McGuire 1982; Bord and Faulkner 1983; Csordas 1994). McGuire began ethnographic research on five Catholic Pentecostal groups in 1971 and expanded her observations to two more groups in 1973 and another two in 1976 and 1977. Csordas (1994) conducted ethnographic research among Catholic charismatics in southeastern New England. His sample included 87 healers and 587 participants who attended large public healing services conducted by five of these healers.

McGuire characterizes Catholic charismatics as "middle-class, moderately well-educated, and generally not the 'type' social scientists would expect to be attracted to an alternative medical system" (1982:128). She reported that her subjects' views of biomedicine ranged from dissatisfaction to anger. Many of the people she interviewed were attracted to a wide array of alternative medical practices, including chiropractic, natural foods, and mega-therapy (McGuire 1982:141–42). In a sample of 508 participants who attended large public healing services, anthropologist Thomas Csordas (1994:30) found that 115 (22.6 percent) were professionals, 117 (23.0 percent) were skilled workers,

71 (14.0 percent) were semi-skilled workers, 110 (21.7 percent) were house-wives, and 95 (18.7 percent) were students or retired or unemployed individu-als. Bord and Faulkner (1983:9) reported that in their sample of 987 adherents of the Catholic charismatic movement, 62 percent were female and 38 per-cent were male. The highest level of education attained for 14.3 percent was an advanced degree; 24.9 percent, a college degree; 37.0 percent, some col-lege education; 15.8 percent, a high school diploma; 4.9 percent, some high school education; 1.4 percent, completion of junior high school; 0.8 percent, only a grade school education (Bord and Faulkner 1983:9).

Catholic charismatic services typically last three or four hours if preceded by mass and involve several types of healing. Csordas (1983:336) delineates four types of charismatic healing: physical healing, spiritual healing, the heal-ing of memories, and deliverance. Physical healing is used for specific so-matic ailments and entails laying on of hands accompanied by prayer. Al-though popularized by various Protestant evangelists like Oral Roberts and Katherine Kuhlman, it does not occur very often in Catholic charismatic circles. Spiritual healing is associated with confession and "provides a crucial religious underpinning for Catholic Pentecostal healing, in that it is directly concerned with the well-being of the soul" (Csordas 1983:337). In the heal-ing of memories, or inner healing, the congregation prays for healing from traumatic events that have occurred during the supplicant's life. Deliverance refers to a "form of healing in which the adverse effects of demons or evil spirits on a person's behavior and personality are removed by expulsion of the spirits judged to be responsible" (Csordas 1983:336). In her observations on several Catholic neo-Pentecostal groups, McGuire (1982:142) found the following range of prayer requests: physical healings, 30–50 percent; men-tal healings, 30–40 percent; healing of relationships, 10–30 percent; requests for career advancement or financial security, 5–15 percent; requests for assis-tance in making decisions, 0–5 percent; and general requests, 5–10 percent.

Both McGuire (1982) and Csordas (1994) see the search for empowerment as central to Catholic charismatic healing. McGuire asserts that even rela-tively affluent people in American society "sense that change has 'robbed' them of the power to control the future, to effect their wills on their en-vironment, to know what to expect and to act accordingly" (1982:176). She maintains that, despite the tendency of Catholic charismatics to be politically conservative, the spread of faith healing, including in the context of Catholic neo-Pentecostalism, may "represent a political statement against the power of the medical establishment—especially its monopoly over the definition of deviance and its unwillingness to include spiritual values in the definition of health" (McGuire 1982:183).

Relying upon a phenomenological approach, Csordas views Catholic char-ismatic healing as a means for creating a "sacred self" in American society.

He describes it as a "system of ritual performance" composed of body, mind, and spirit, which mobilizes and organizes self processes (Csordas 1994:26). Ritual healing, unlike the miracle cures often associated with evangelical faith healing, often enables adherents to "operate on a margin of disability that is present in many conditions" (Csordas 1994:498). In the healing of memories, Csordas asserts, the perception of divine presence often instills in Catholic charismatics a sense of security that enables them to overcome memories of traumatic events. It is also possible the Catholic charismatic movement may provide partial empowerment to women by allowing them to serve as healers in the context of patriarchical structures. Indeed, of the 87 healing ministers in Csordas's sample, seven were nuns and 47 were laywomen.

DIANETICS AND SCIENTOLOGY

L. Ron Hubbard's *Dianetics: The Modern Science of Mental Health* (1950) served as the foundation for what Hubbard (1911–1986) initially regarded as an alternative form of psychotherapy (Wallis 1977). He believed that the Reactive Mind is an elaborate computer containing the potential of total recall of all sense impressions. Painful past experiences are stored in the subconscious mind as "engrams" and prevent people from functioning to the fullest of their capacities. Hubbard referred to the individual who had achieved a state of vastly improved mental agility as a "clear." In 1952 Hubbard established the Hubbard Research Foundation in Elizabeth, New Jersey, but moved it to Wichita, Kansas, and later to Phoenix, Arizona. He formed the Founding Church of Scientology in Washington, D.C., in 1954 and the Hubbard College of Scientology at Saint Hill in Sussex, England, in 1959.

Hubbard eventually became disenchanted with his lack of control over the organizational fissioning of Dianetics. In 1952 he claimed to have received new revelations and insights that transformed Dianetics into the sectarian religion of Scientology. According to Ellwood,

> Scientology was different from Dianetics in at least two respects: the concept of the thetan and the E-meter. The thetan is the individual consciousness, which Hubbard said has the capacity to separate from the body and mind, and to create MEST—matter, energy, space, and time. To be Clear is to understand more fully how one is a spiritual being or a thetan, and thereby to gain control over one's mind and physical environment. (1973:170)

Development of the E-meter (E for engram) was an attempt to provide scientific credibility. A counselor or auditor would question a client about his past life while holding a tin can wired to a needle that purportedly detected sensitive topics. Hubbard had a new revelation about reincarnation that called for the need to eliminate engrams not only from one's present life but also from one's previous lives, thereby lengthening the healing process. Scientology teaches that many psychosomatic ailments are the result of the thetan being out of communication with a particular part of the body. Scientology denies that it is a system of physical healing, but rather claims that it is concerned with the improvement of intelligence, personal growth, and success. Bromley and Bracey see the Church of Scientology as "one of the clearest examples of a quasi-religious therapy system" (1998:152).

Hubbard created an elaborate hierarchy of release grades and levels of auditors. The 1982 booklet "From Clear to Eternity" listed 64 release grades (Stark and Bainbridge 1985:276). Hubbard also developed numerous mental exercises designed to assist clients in releasing engrams, with the ultimate goal of becoming a clear. This process was very costly:

> In mid-1979, the Los Angeles org [organization] was charging $3,692.87 for the solo audit course, $1,777.84 for the grade IV release that followed it, and $2,844.54 for the clearing course. Solo assists, if done separately from the solo audit course, cost $923.22 for those individuals who sought this help. Among the most expensive special aids, New Era Dianetics, offered to clears, was sold at about $250 an hour. . . The org offers package deals, and, in mid-1979, 50 hours of New Era Dianetics suitable for clears was available for a straight price of $12,603.61. (Stark and Bainbridge 1985:272)

Zellner (1995:103) characterizes Scientology as a "hard-sell, money-gouging, high stakes enterprise" which prompts its adherents to enroll in numerous courses in order to become clear.

The Church of Scientology is organized into over 1,000 churches, missions, and related organizations in 74 countries, which provide introductory training, and it claims to have over 10,000 staff members (Bromley and Bracey 1998:154). The "mother church" in Los Angeles sets standards for branch organizations, monitors their activities, and offers advanced training. Over two-thirds of current members are reportedly between the ages of 20 and 40 (Bromley and Bracey 1998:149). The Church reports that the vast majority of its members are white-collar workers and that nearly 15 percent own their own businesses. It also claims that about 17,000 practitioners had attained the status of clear by 1980, and that nearly 50,000 had done so by 1995.

Scientology has actively championed the rights of mental patients. It has provoked controversy in the United States and other countries by attacking the U.S. Internal Revenue Service and the psychiatric profession, particularly for its reliance upon electric shock treatment and psychotropic drugs such as Ritalin and Proszac (Bednarowski 1995:390).

Wallis (1977:245) characterizes Scientology as a manipulationist movement that provides a perspective for explaining a person's situation and a set of procedures for improving his or her condition. In keeping with its overwhelmingly middle-class membership, it provides a "religious commodity eminently suited to the contemporary market" (Wallis 1977:247). Like the New Thought groups, Scientology attempts to provide its adherents with metaphysical solutions that will enable them to achieve success in the existing social order — one in which many individuals experience a lack of control over their lives. Wallis asserts that, in keeping with organizational life in the larger society, "communication within the movement is relatively impersonal; relationships are role-articulated; and the organization is bureaucratic" (1977:245). In contrast, Stark and Bainbridge (1985:281) found Scientology to be "well-designed to provide a rich supply of individual attention and affect to newcomers" within the context of a religious congregation.

The religious healing systems discussed in this chapter reflect both class and gender aspects of Anglo-American social life in the United States. Whereas Christian Science and, more recently, Scientology, tend to appeal largely to upper-middle-class individuals, Spiritualism, Unity, and perhaps other New Thought healing systems have tended to cater by and large to lower-middle-class individuals. Furthermore, in contrast to Pentecostalism, which initially found its greatest appeal among working-class people — including, as the next chapter indicates, African Americans — the charismatic movement, or neo-Pentecostalism, both mainstream denominations and evangelical sects, has tended to cater to socially upwardly mobile individuals. Except perhaps for Scientology, women have tended to occupy the role of religious healer within Spiritualism, Christian Science, other New Thought groups, and Pentecostalism.

8

Folk Medical Systems in a Culturally Diverse Society

Despite the preeminence of biomedicine, folk medical systems persist and even thrive in the United States. This chapter focuses on folk medicine among several ethnic groups: European Americans, African Americans, Haitian Americans, Latinos or Hispanic Americans, Asian Americans, and Native Americans.

In contrast to the medical systems found among people of color, European American ethnomedicine exhibits both a professionalized sector and a folk sector. The professionalized sector of European American ethnomedicine includes biomedicine; osteopathic medicine, a parallel medical system; and chiropractic and naturopathy, professionalized heterodox medical systems. Acupuncture has been quickly evolving into a full-fledged professionalized heterodox medical system even though its philosophical and therapeutic roots of acupuncture are Chinese and, to a lesser degree, Japanese. As acupuncture accommodates itself to biomedicine and Western science, it is assuming an increasingly European American cast. European American ethnomedicine also includes an array of partially professionalized medical systems situated along a continuum between the professional and folk sectors, some of which are contained under the umbrella of the holistic health movement, as well as several religious healing systems that were the focus of the previous chapter. Finally, it includes regional folk medical systems such as southern Appalachian herbal medicine and those of the "Pennsylvania Dutch."

While providing a brief overview of European American regional folk medicine, this chapter focuses primarily on folk medical systems among people of color in the United States. Like indigenous medical systems or the medical systems of peasant peoples, the folk medical systems of ethnic groups in the United States invariably include religious components. It is important to note that people of color often resort to European American ethnomedicine, particularly in its professionalized and religious forms, whereas European Americans only occasionally seek out folk and religious healers associated with various ethnic minorities. The imbalance in this pattern of

144

dual use attests to the persisting racist and ethnocentric nature of American society. European American folk medicine and the folk medical systems found among people of color have not existed in isolation but have influenced each other. Regardless of the ethnic group, folk medical systems thrive for the most part among working-class people, many of whom constitute the poorest, most economically exploited, politically oppressed, socially stigmatized, and discriminated-against segments of American society.

EUROPEAN AMERICAN FOLK MEDICINE

The folk sector of European ethnomedicine includes southern Appalachian and Ozark herbal medicine and the folk medical systems of the Mormons in the Intermountain West and of Anabaptist groups such as the Amish and Mennonites residing in Pennsylvania and several midwestern states (e.g., Ohio, Indiana, Iowa, and Wisconsin) and the Hutterites of the northern Plains states. European American folk medicine is not a homogenous system but rather a diverse array of localized medical systems that represent many different European countries and time periods. It was heavily shaped by the frontier experience and influenced by Native American healing systems and also, particularly in the South, by African American folk medicine. Although European American folk medicine constitutes a legitimate topic of research for both anthropologists and sociologists, it has tended to be primarily a concern of folklorists. Foster and Anderson observe that European American folk medicine emerged to a large extent as a phenomenon related to high literacy rates:

> It was in the United States where, for the first time in history, the great majority of people who depended on their own resources and those of the local curer could read. And read they did; it was a rare family that did not, along with its bible, carry with it one or more home remedy books and read in local newspapers the extravagant, usually fraudulent, claims made by local "doctors" and patent medicines. (1978:71)

APPALACHIAN HERBAL MEDICINE

European American folk medicine has a more significant presence in the southern than in the northern United States. In their overview of Appalachian herbal medicine, Evans, Kileff, and Shelley (1982) assert that a "significantly high portion of the Appalachian population" utilized it at one time or another. Based upon interviews with 63 practitioners who resided within a 50-mile radius of Chattanooga, Tennessee, they identified four types of herbalists:

the "family therapist," the "practitioner specialist," the "professional herbalist," and the "institutional herbalist." Fifty of the practitioners were family herbalists. These herbalists were highly individualistic and tended to rely on a limited number of herbs, knowledge of which had been passed down from generation to generation in certain families. In part as a result of their strong antagonism toward biomedical physicians and the tradition of rugged individualism characteristic of Appalachian mountain folk, family herbalists emphasize the self-help approach to most aspects of health care. The work of Icy, a retired school teacher who received her knowledge of herbs from her grandfather and mother as well as from a number of books, exemplifies that of the practitioner specialist. In contrast to the straightforward method of the family therapist, who applies a single herb for a particular illness, the practitioner specialist combines several herbs as well as non-herbal substances and regards his or her methods as complementary to those of biomedicine. Doctors Caldwell and Fields were two well-known professional herbalists who operated clinics in a small town. While both of them were secretive about their methods and antagonistic toward biomedicine, they differed in impression management and in the types of clients they attracted. Doctor Caldwell's folksy office drew a generally older group of patients from a large area, including several nearby states; in contrast, Doctor Fields's work setting resembled that of an M.D. in both appearance and equipment, consequently attracting younger, more urban patients from the immediate area. Institutional herbalists worked in settings such as the Wildwood Sanitarium and Hospital, a Seventh-day Adventist institution located outside of Chattanooga.

Stekert (1970) reported on the persistence of the following southern Appalachian folk medical beliefs and practices among female migrants to Detroit: a general hostility or indifference toward biomedical physicians; a glorification of folk healers (particularly older women); and the tendency among women to return home for care when they were either seriously sick or pregnant. Although southern Appalachian migrants to midwestern cities continue to use folk medical practices, Cavender and Beck, in their study of folk medicine in and around Hiltons, a rural community in southwestern Virginia, reported that the "1920s and 1930s mark the time when a dependence on botanicals was on the decline in many communities throughout the region"(1995:134).

OTHER EUROPEAN AMERICAN FOLK MEDICAL SYSTEMS

European American folk medicine continues to persist in rural communities not only in the South but also in the Middle Atlantic states, the Midwest, and the Intermountain West (Roebuck and Quan 1976). Carl Withers reported the existence of "five historical layers of medical and pseudomedical lore" in Smalltown (pseudonym), a small midwestern town: "(1) Early magical practice, including both 'witchcraft' and divine healing; (2) an enormous body of 'home remedies'; (3) rational or pseudo-rational medicine connected with the recognized medical profession; (4) patent medicines; and (5) a new and recent wave of curing by prayer and other religious techniques" (1946:234).

Although the Amish do not reject biomedicine on biblical grounds, they continue to subscribe to a distinctive ethnomedical system of their own that incorporates remedies along with the use of magical charms and other supernatural practices (Hostetler 1976).

Several German Protestant groups and other European American groups use a technique called "powwowing," in which the healer whispers prayers or biblical verses into the ear of a client, often accompanied by laying on of hands (Yoder 1966). Some powwowers utilize one or a few traditional charms in order to remove warts or stop blood.

"Talking fire out of burns" is a healing technique that has been traced back to medieval Europe and has been documented among both European Americans and African Americans in some sections of the United States, including the Ozarks, Louisiana, Indiana, Illinois, Pennsylvania, Michigan, and parts of the Southeast (Kirkland 1992:41). A burn healer treats a burn by praying and manipulating a charm in order to summon supernatural forces. Some burn healers apply various substances to the surface of the burn while performing their magical-religious procedures.

AFRICAN AMERICAN FOLK MEDICINE

African American folk medicine developed within the context of North American slavery. African peoples sought the protection of their gods and ancestral spirits and relied upon charms and medicinal plants in dealing with the uncertainties of life and death. They turned to priests, diviners, mediums, and healers who served as intermediaries between themselves and the supernatural realm. Cross-fertilization among the health beliefs and practices of blacks, whites, and American Indians occurred during the antebellum period in the rural South. The terms *conjure, rootwork,* and *hoodoo* came to be applied to an elaborate system of health care, magic, divination, herbalism, and witchcraft widespread among African American slaves. Raboteau views conjure as the "symbolized translation of African sacred charms into Afro-American magical medicine" (1986:548). Many conjurers were skilled herbalists and adept observers of human relationships.

The slaves and their descendants also drew upon Christianity for comprehending illness and misfortune. They came to regard illness as the will of God, the malevolence of the devil, or punishment for sin. The slaves were able to discover elements in Christianity that were consistent with their own aspi-

147

rations for freedom and experience-shaped perception of reality. The slaves did not unilaterally accept the cosmology of the whites. Rather, as Levine notes, "for the slave, Heaven and Hell were not [abstract] concepts but places which could be experienced during one's lifetime; God and Christ and Satan were not symbols but personages with whom meetings or confrontations were quite possible" (1977:37). Although heaven might indeed at times be construed in otherworldly terms, it might also be viewed, depending on the context, as Africa, Jerusalem, Canada, or some other sought-after earthly sanctuary. Jesus was a knowable helper and healer who approached humans as imperfect beings rather than as condemned sinners. In constructing a theology of hope, the slaves preserved their sense of identity and dignity while resisting the psychological trauma of an oppressive social system. While the Baptist and Methodist churches to which African Americans flocked during both the antebellum and the post–Civil War era expressed criticism of mediums and diviners, these roles reappeared in the Holiness-Pentecostal and Spiritual sects of the early twentieth century.

In essence, African American folk medicine became a diverse ensemble drawing upon different cultural traditions:

> The system is a composite of the classical medicine of an earlier day, European folklore regarding the natural world, rare African traits, and selected beliefs derived from modern scientific medicine. The whole is inextricably blended with tenets of fundamentalist Christianity, elements from the Voodoo religions of the West Indies, and the added spice of sympathetic magic. . . . It is a coherent medical system and not a ragtag collection of isolated superstitions. (Snow 1974:83)

Folk practices continue to be a vital part of health care delivery for African Americans in both the rural South and the cities of the South and the North. Many working-class African Americans rely on home remedies and folk practitioners. African American folk medicine combines both naturalistic and personalistic theories of disease etiology (Snow 1977). Health in African American culture is viewed as the "ability to 'keep on keepin' on" and the harmony of body, mind, and spirit (Snow 1993:73). Blood plays a central role in African American folk medicine and may be regarded as "too high" or "too low" in volume, "too thick" or "too thin" in consistency, too "pure" or "impure," and as "shooting too high" or "falling too low" in the body (Snow 1993: 99).

Contemporary African American folk healers can be divided into four main types: independent generalists, independent specialists, cultic generalists, and cultic specialists (Baer 1982). As this typology indicates, healers may or not affiliate their healing practices with a religious group or congregation. I use the term *independent healers* to refer to healers who operate as individuals or are affiliated with some sort of occult supply store, either as owner, employee, or renter, and *cultic healers* to refer to those affiliated with a religious group. Whereas independent healers function exclusively or almost exclusively in private settings, cultic healers may practice in both public and private settings. Certain individuals function in both capacities, either compartmentalizing or mixing the two modes of practice. An excellent example of this pattern is described in Winslow's (1969) case study of Bishop E. E. Everett and his occult store in Philadelphia. Bishop Everett was the pastor of and a healer in the Calvary Spiritual Temple, a congregation affiliated with the Apostolic Church of Christ in God, headquartered in Martinville, Virginia. He was also the proprietor of the Calvary Religious and Occult Store, an enterprise not located in the church. Bishop Everett sold a variety of magico-religious articles and gave advice on them to a largely working-class African American and Puerto Rican clientele, but "many members of his congregation [were] persons whom he contacted when they came to his store to make purchases or seek spiritual advice" (Winslow 1969:63). Both independent and cultic *generalists* treat a wide array of complications of both a psychosocial and physical nature; independent and cultic *specialists* focus on particular ailments or employ specific modalities, such as prescribing herbs or religious articles.

INDEPENDENT GENERALISTS

The central character in African American folk medicine historically has been the *conjurer,* who also goes under other labels, including *conjure doctor, rootworker, hoodoo doctor,* and *hungan.* Whitten (1962:315–16) describes the conjurer as a "professional diviner, curer, agent finder, and general controller of the occult arts." Conjurers reputedly possess one or more traits that distinguish them from ordinary mortals. These include "double-sight," or the ability to see ghosts, being born on Christmas, being a seventh son, or a having an atypical physical trait such as albinism, dwarfism, green eyes, or three birthmarks on the left arm (Bass 1981:381). Individuals become conjurers in one of three ways: inheritance of the position, apprenticeship under the tutelage of an established practitioner, or a "calling" from God.

The conjurer's most important functions are to cure people who have been bewitched—that is, "conjured," "fixed," "crossed," or "hexed"—and to place a direct spell or counterspell upon the client's enemies. Conjurers also concern themselves with a large number of other conditions, ranging from somatic ailments to problems of everyday life. Clients seek out conjurers for success in business or financial endeavors, gambling, and obtaining gainful employment; resolution of strained social relations with significant others; the search for a spouse; avoidance of the law; a favorable decision in court; control over superordinates, such as a landlord or employer; and discovery of unknown enemies. Clients also turn to conjurers to tell their fortunes or to cure physical ailments. In attempting to solve their clients' problems, conjurers generally prescribe a variety of items, including perfumes, oils, seeds, powders, roots, pictures of Catholic saints, candles, medals, and readings from the Bible or the sixth and seventh Books of Moses.

With the mass migration of African Americans to cities in both the North and the South, hoodoo or conjure became incorporated and transformed into new forms, such as Spiritualism and commercialism. Cooley (1977:193) contends that the new guise of conjurers as "psychics," "spiritualistic readers," and "prophets" was a move toward respectability and legal protection. Hurston (1931:319) notes that hoodoo was often blended with Spiritualism in New Orleans in order to provide hoodoo doctors with a protective screen from legal prosecution. Although many Spiritualists and psychics claim to be ministers, in reality they often function as independent healers who are willing to treat a wide number of problems and concerns. Spiritualists may be affiliated in some capacity with an occult supply store or operate on a strictly individual basis. In time, they may convert their practice into a religious congregation, perhaps using some of their clients as the group's core membership. In contrast to conjurers and rootworkers, who make extensive use of roots and herbs in attempting to gain control over the hidden forces of the universe, Spiritualists tend to have limited knowledge of these substances and are more likely to use them in the form of baths and teas. Many Spiritualists advertise in African American newspapers, magazines, and on radio stations (Snow 1978).

INDEPENDENT SPECIALISTS

Probably the best known independent specialists are herbalists or rootworkers in the strict sense of the word. Herbalists specialize in applying medicinal plants and other remedies for common ailments. Mr. Lee, an herbalist in Louisiana, utilized medicinal plants found in Chatham and Lee counties in North Carolina (Payne-Jackson and Lee 1993:27). Although herbalists are most common in rural areas, undoubtedly because of the ready availability of medicinal plants, Hall and Bourne (1973:138–39) mentioned three people, two men and one woman, who operated herb shops in the Price neighborhood of Atlanta. Watson (1984:60) found an increase in the use of medicinal plants as clients' incomes increased from $1,000 to $2,000–3,000 per year, but a decrease with incomes above $3,000.

Female neighborhood practitioners, who are closely related to herbalists, are often referred to by terms such as "Old Lady," "granny," or "Mrs. Markus." The Old Lady is essentially a local consultant on common ailments. She does not have office hours or dispense medicine per se but merely advises clients on how to treat ordinary illnesses. Although she may occasionally receive monetary compensation for her services, she is more likely to receive an expression of gratitude or a gift of food. A subtype of the Old Lady is the "granny" midwife, a black woman who works under the informal supervision of a biomedical physician (Dougherty 1982). Commenting on the rural county in North Carolina where they did research on granny midwives, Mongeau, Smith, and Maney (1961:504) assert that African American midwifery constituted an "active" but "restless and uncertain" endeavor, particularly because there were no longer apprentice midwives in the area. The decline of granny midwifery is also indicated by the fact that whereas midwives performed 67.4 percent of all recorded "nonwhite" deliveries and 11.4 percent of all white deliveries in 1936 in North Carolina, by 1966 they performed only 23.6 percent of "nonwhite" deliveries and a small fraction of one percent of white deliveries (Mongeau, Smith, and Maney 1961:497). Mathews (1992) interprets the disappearance of the granny midwife in North Carolina as having stemmed in large part from restrictive legislation that pushed them out of practice. The biomedical establishment and state health agencies discriminated against granny midwives, who, as poor black women, were members of a triple minority.

An important source of advice for some African Americans in their quest for health, love, economic success, and satisfactory interpersonal relationships is the "magic vendor" (Hall and Bourne 1973). Magic vendors are owners or employees of commercial enterprises that sell occult articles. Although probably most of the small and medium-sized occult stores (often referred as "candle stores") are owned by blacks, many of the large stores are owned by whites, as apparently are the companies that manufacture the articles that are sold in them. Some regular drugstores in ghetto areas also stock occult items.

CULTIC GENERALISTS

The term cultic generalist refers to Spiritual advisors, Voodoo priests, and black Islamic and Hebraic healers who treat a variety of illnesses either within the context of religious services or in private consultations. Voodoo priests and priestesses serve as important religious functionaries in temples. They not only conduct ceremonies in honor of the African gods (*loa*) but also engage in healing, divination, and evidently—at least occasionally—sorcery. During the eighteenth century, slaves were brought to Louisiana from Africa and from the Caribbean islands of Martinique, Guadeloupe, and Saint Domingue (now Haiti). Although Voodoo was probably imported into Louisiana with slaves from the islands, its principal introduction into the region apparently occurred later, in the early nineteenth century, when French masters escaping the revolution in Saint Domingue brought slaves with them, and free blacks arrived as refugees. During the nineteenth century, Voodoo meetings—presided over by "queens" and "witch doctors"—catered to slaves, free blacks, and some white women (Reinders 1961:241). As a result of anti-Voodoo sentiment among whites and legal actions that began about 1820 and surfaced periodically during the nineteenth century, Voodoo in New Orleans was forced to go into hiding. However, in recent decades Voodoo, or *vodun*, has undergone a revitalization in the United States as a result of the migration of Haitians to southern Florida, New York, and other urban areas (Brown 1991)—a subject discussed later in the chapter.

Anthropologist Loudell Snow conducted ethnographic research on Mother D, a Voodoo practitioner in a southwestern city. Mother D identified herself as a *mambo* and claimed that she had inherited her power from her maternal grandmother (Snow 1973:277). She held a ministerial license and a Doctor of Divinity degree from the International Universal Church and maintained a religious healing complex consisting of two stucco buildings in a Mexican American barrio, about a mile from a predominantly African American neighborhood:

> The larger of the buildings, an old house, contains a store where oils, incenses and religious items may be purchased, a small chapel, and the home of her son, Fred G, and his wife. The chapel is a curious combination of Roman Catholic, African, and zodiacal elements. The altar table holds votive candles, a large portrait of St. Theresa of the Little Flower, the Infant Jesus of Prague, a Pyrex bowl of water, and a large, jointed, wooden snake. Sticks of incense burn in holes in the snake's back. . . . the snake is a symbol of the African serpent God, Damballah Ouedo, of West Africa and Haiti. (Snow 1978:89–90)

Mother D conducted regular services on Sunday mornings and Friday evenings. While most of the members of her congregation were African Americans, her clients were mostly Mexican Americans along with some Native Americans or Anglos. Mother D treated her clients in the smaller building. Her examining room contained a hospital bed, a chair, a small table covered with bottles and jars, and statues of the Virgin Mary and various saints. Fred G also had an office where he administered massages, prescribed herbs and other medicinal substances, and gave advice. Mother D reported that most of her clients suffered from "nervousness." She also treated clients who believed that they had been bewitched and claimed that people could bewitch themselves. Mother D maintained that she could cure cancers, tumors, arthritis, and other "natural" illnesses by laying on of hands. She also provided advice for problems of living and administered herbal teas and massages.

Spiritual prophets, also known as advisors or mediums, many of whom are women, function within the context of the highly syncretic Spiritual movement, which combines elements from American Spiritualism, Roman Catholicism, African American Protestantism, and Voodoo as well as other systems, such as New Thought, Islam, Judaism, and/or astrology (Baer 1984a; Jacobs and Kaslow 1991). Spiritual prophets claim to possess a gift from the Spirit which enables them to prophesy and heal (Baer 1981a; Jacobs 1990). Although they may treat physical ailments, Spiritual prophets tend to focus on the socioeconomic and psychosocial problems that poor blacks in particular, but also middle-class and non-poor working-class blacks as well as some white clients, encounter in everyday life. Spiritual prophets often direct messages concerning the past, present, and future to specific individuals during the course of religious services, particularly those known as as "bless services" or "prophesy services." They also provide private consultations for their clients. In addition to the "reading" or message from the Spirit, Spiritual prophets say prayers or recite scriptural passages or provide magico-religious rituals, roots, and herbs for their clients.

Some, if not most, messianic-nationalist sects, such as African American Muslim and Judaic groups, appear to have healers of some sort (Baer and Singer 1992). Singer (1981) discusses the role of religious healing in the social system of the Original Hebrew Israelite Nation, a group with African American congregations in both the United States and Israel. Unlike in many African American Holiness-Pentecostal and Spiritual groups, divine healing among the Black Hebrews consists of a fully developed and exclusive set of beliefs about disease causation and a related regimen of treatment procedures. The chief healer or "Rofa" in the Nation's community in Israel was a middle-aged woman who had assumed this role during the group's interim settlement in Liberia. She was assisted by a staff of "nurses" and trained other divine healers. According to Singer, the "Rofa serves both as a somatic healer and psychotherapist for the Black Hebrew community" (1981:218). While she devoted much of her time to the delivery of infants, she also attended to a variety of physical ailments and listened to the personal problems of members of the community.

CULTIC SPECIALISTS

Cultic specialists are faith healers who tend to focus on psychosomatic ailments within a religious setting. Both African American Holiness-Pentecostal ("Sanctified") and Spiritual churches have religious healers, often referred to as "divine healers," who claim to possess the gift of healing, but who may lack the gift of prophecy. Black divine healers use diverse techniques, including laying on of hands, anointing with oil, using blessed water, and applying prayer cloths to the sick body. According to Raboteau, Sanctified churches foster health by requiring their members to "refrain from tobacco, alcohol, narcotics, gambling, and 'worldly' amusements" (1986:555).

African American evangelical faith healers generally are pastors or prominent members of religious congregations. Despite the fact that evangelical faith healers may constitute the largest single category of folk therapists in African American communities, relatively little has been written about them. Hall and Bourne (1973:139) note that healing in their services generally is used as "a mechanism to underscore some message of the teaching and as evidence of the validity of their promising good times on this earth" if that teaching is followed. Some variation of laying on of hands appears to be the most commonly employed healing technique used by faith healers. They also anoint with holy oil and give their clients prayer cloths and blessed waters. Although it does not appear that most evangelical faith healers do "readings," many offer advice to clients on how to solve problems of living.

THE CONTRADICTORY NATURE OF
AFRICAN AMERICAN FOLK MEDICINE

Like African American religion, to which it is strongly related, African American folk medicine juxtaposes elements of protest and accommodation (Baer and Singer 1992). In the past, whites feared the conjurer, whom they regarded as the Devil's secret agent. Genovese (1974:222) maintains that, despite a sense of empowerment that conjurers gave slaves, ultimately conjurers were "accommodationists" who were unable to affect the balance of power. In contrast to Genovese, David Brown views conjure as a multivalent force that did more than provide comfort to its clients, even after Emancipation:

> After slavery conjure continued to serve a subtle counterhegemonic role—at least to the extent that in reported cases it subverted white expectations of black behavior and labor productivity. Conjure was regularly used, moreover, as an effective weapon—it was claimed—to subvert prosecution of blacks in court. It often effectively prevented the prosecutor from "talking" or prevented the judge from finding or using court "papers." (1990:35)

Conjure serves as the prototype for other variants of African American folk medicine. Within the context of the Spiritual movement, prophets and advisors function as folk therapists who are well acquainted with (and communicate a genuine concern about) the problems of their clients. It is possible that the techniques used by these prophets and advisors enable clients, at least to some extent, to overcome a state of demoralization. A common theme in the Spiritual movement is the notion that one has to think positively and overcome negative modes of thought. Prophets and advisors constantly remind their clients that they must believe in themselves, and that if they do not, no one else will. For the most part, they focus on individualistic concerns—a trend that is in keeping with the increasing privatization that characterizes much of modern life, particularly in urban areas. Consequently, the complex of prophets and advisors has a hegemonic dimension in that it tends to deny "political conflict by stressing the importance of individual over society, the insignificance of social arrangements and plans, and the irrelevance of group conflict beside the paramount importance of the individual" (Wilson 1978: 356). Spiritual advisors inadvertently "blame the victim" by overlooking the social and economic roots of many of their clients' problems. They promise their clients improvements in their lives if they engage in certain magico-religious rituals, develop a positive attitude, and overcome negative thoughts.

In addition to providing a form of health care that is often cheaper than biomedicine, African American folk medicine serves as a significant source of cultural identity and pride. It has evolved from African-based syncretic religions like Voodoo in southern Louisiana during the nineteenth century to a variety of forms: conjure, rootwork, or hoodoo in slave communities and present-day rural areas of the South; religious healing practices based primarily in Sanctified (Holiness-Pentecostal) and Spiritual churches; and, most recently, the practices of highly visible religious or psychic healers such as the Reverend Ike, who promises his adherents "Green Power," and Dione Warwick, who appears in television commercials advertising the services of the "Psychic Connection"—a capitalistic venture. As Semmes observes, "Southern, rural, and small town migrants, and others carried health-related magico-religious beliefs with them large cities, which became important but not dominant variants of traditional healing practices" (1996:79). Another indication of the process of assimilation manifested in African American health practices is the growing interest on the part of some African Americans in heterodox medical systems like naturopathy and chiropractic (Semmes 1996: 89–103).

FOLK MEDICINE AMONG HAITIAN AMERICANS

Most Haitian Americans came to the United States during the administrations of François Duvalier (ruled 1957–1971) and his son, Jean-Claude, who succeeded him in 1971. Although they are found in almost every state, the majority of Haitian Americans are concentrated in large cities such as New York, Miami, Boston, Chicago, and Washington, D.C. Haitian American communities generally have their own churches, stores, restaurants, social and literary clubs, newspapers, and folk healers.

Haitian Americans, most of whom are working class but some of whom are middle class, often continue to use home remedies in addition to frequenting biomedical physicians, clinics, and hospitals. Laguerre asserts that Haitian Americans exhibit diverse patterns of health care behavior "as a result of differences in their past medical experience, their previous class status in Haiti, and their immigrant status in the United States" (1984:108). Traditional Haitian Americans categorize illnesses into natural illnesses, known as *maladi pei* (country diseases) or *maladi bon die* (diseases of the Lord), and supernatural illnesses, which are attributed to the angry spirits.

Voodoo, which is known by a variety of terms (including *vodun, vodu, vandoux,* and *vaudou*), is the primary form of religious healing among both Haitians and Haitian Americans. The term *vodun,* meaning "god," comes from Dahomey and serves as a generic term for all the deities or *loa*. As Herskovits observes, "*vodun* is neither the practice of black magic, nor the unorganized pathological hysteria it is often represented to be" (1971:153). Voodoo is essentially the folk religion of the Haitian people; it is a syncretic ensemble that blends together elements of West African religion and Roman Catholicism. The loa tend to be associated with various Catholic saints — either as one and the same, as separate but mutually cooperative spirits, or as antagonistic beings. Among the loa, Azaka is a peasant who portrays poverty and the ravaged soil of Haiti; Ogou is a warrior who represents the harsh lessons of Haitian history; Kouzinn is the female counterpart of Azaka and a symbol of Haitian gender politics; and Ezili represents a collectivity of female attributes such as empowerment, hard work, and sensuality (Brown 1991).

Voodoo includes beliefs and rituals directed at the loa and specialists who serve as intermediaries between believers and the spirits. Male Voodoo priests (*houngans*) and female Voodoo priests (*mambos*) conduct ceremonies in honor of the loa and ancestral spirits and function as cultic healers. Voodoo places of worship serve as religious healing centers. Whereas they often are situated in temples in Haiti, religious healing centers tend to be situated in single rooms and basements in the United States (Laguerre 1984:59). During the healing process, the loa "mount a horse," or possess a devotee, and demand sacrifices for their sustenance. According to Murphy (1994:37), the loa are "called to a specific role in balancing the never-ending imbalances" of the poor. Devotees do not remember having been possessed. Voodoo priests mediate between the devotee and the supernatural realm by divining which spirit must be appeased. The spirit informs the devotee what he or she must do to recover and which medication to take after the proper ritual duties have been conducted.

Karen McCarthy Brown (1991) wrote a "thick" ethnographic account of Alourdes, a mambo who performed religious healing rituals on both an individual basis and a collective basis in her Brooklyn home. Alourdes practiced a healing art that had passed through at least three generations of her family. She was one of several hundred mambos who ministered to Haitian immigrants in New York City. After spending her twenties in Port-au-Prince, she came to Brooklyn in 1962, and shortly thereafter sent for her three children, including Maggie, who also became a *mambo*. Alourdes's mother, Philo, often assisted her in her practice by appearing in her dreams. Alourdes obtained her healing power primarily from Gede, the spirit of death. Through her ritual prescriptions, Alourdes attempted to provide her clients with survival skills — not only ritualistic ones, but also those that conferred a sense of self-respect that would enable them to deal with the hardships of their lives.

As other observers of Voodoo such as Zora Neale Hurston (1931) and Alfred Metraux (1972) have noted, Voodoo is a pragmatic religion that focuses on the concrete problems of everyday life. Brown maintains that Voodoo serves as "the repository for wisdom accumulated by a people who have lived through slavery, hunger, disease, repression, corruption, and violence — all in excess" (1991:98). Although she does not explain how Alourdes overcame the vissici-tudes of abject poverty, it is clear that Alourdes's work as a Voodoo healer gave her sufficient financial resources to purchase her own home and to support, along with her daughter's outside income, a three-generation family. Brown contends that Voodoo has empowered women more than the great majority of religions have and provides its adherents with an important coping mecha-nism in situations where revolution appears to be impossible. It is a pragmatic religious healing system with a strong temporal orientation in its emphasis upon the acquisition of health, love, economic prosperity, and interpersonal power.

In addition to Voodoo priests, other religious healers exist among Haitian Americans. Scott (1974) and her co-workers at the University of Miami Health Ecology Project identified two men who identified themselves as "spiritual doctors" and relied upon the Holy Spirit in treating their clients. They also identified five "readers" who divined by reading cards and hands, prophesied, and healed.

FOLK MEDICINE AMONG HISPANIC AMERICANS

Latinos, or Hispanic Americans, comprise many different ethnic groups, in-cluding Mexican Americans, Puerto Ricans, Cuban Americans, Central Americans, and South Americans. While there is some overlap and cross-fertilization among the ethnomedical systems of various groups, each of these systems is distinct. This section discusses *curanderismo* and spiritism among Mexican Americans, *espiritismo* among Puerto Ricans, and *santeria* among Cuban Americans.

CURANDERISMO AMONG MEXICAN AMERICANS

Mexican Americans are concentrated in the Southwest (Texas, New Mexico, Arizona, Colorado, and California) but increasingly are found in other parts of the United States, including the Midwest, the Northeast, and the Southeast. *Curanderismo* constitutes the principal Mexican American folk medical system; the term derives from the Spanish word *curandero* (male) or *curandera* (female) for curer or healer. It has been the focus of considerable anthropological and folkloristic research both in Mexico and the United States (Clark 1970; Rubel 1966; Kay 1977, 1978; Trotter and Chavira 1981; Kay 1993; Koss-Chioino and Canive 1993).

Trotter and Chavira delineate six "major historical influences" that have shaped curanderismo, at least in the Lower Rio Grande Valley. These include: "Judeo-Christian religious beliefs, symbols, and rituals; early Arabic medicine and health practices (combined with Greek humoral medicine, revived during the Spanish Renaissance); medieval and later European witchcraft; Native American herbal lore and health practices; modern beliefs about spiritualism and psychic phenomena; and scientific medicine" (Trotter and Chavira 1981:25). The Bible has influenced curanderismo through reference to the healing properties of animals, plants, oil, and wine; divine intervention; Christ's healing ministry; and the concept of soul. Hispano-Arabic medicine contributed the notions that health constitutes a balanced state and that animals and plants contain curative properties. Curanderismo incorporated a belief in witchcraft or sorcery historically widespread in European and European American cultures. Native American healing systems had a strong impact on curanderismo in terms of the use of medicinal plants and the belief in witchcraft. Curanderismo has been influenced by European spiritism, including the writings of Léon Denizarth Hippolyte Rivail, a French spiritist philosopher better known as Allan Kardec, and now coexists with Mexican and Mexican American espiritismo or spiritism. Finally, curandera/os have adopted several standard biomedical beliefs and practices, including the use of injection drugs.

Mexican American folk medicine classifies illness according to etiology rather than symptoms, distinguishing between two major categories of illness: "natural" ones that result from an imbalance in the divine order, and bewitchments performed by humans who invoke malevolent forces (Madsen 1973:73). Traditional Mexican Americans rely heavily upon medicinal plants. In her ethnographic research in the Sal si Puedes barrio of San Jose, Margaret Clark observed that "almost every kitchen garden has a few plants whose leaves, flowers, or roots are used in the preparation of herb medicines" (1970: 167). Popular medicinal herbs include alfalfa, sweet basil, camphor seeds and leaves, lavender, cinnamon bark, cascara bark, apricot, coriander, cloves, cumin, cassia, dill, saltwort, larkspur, fennel, lemon leaves, orange blossoms, wild marjoram, penny-royal, rosemary, rose of Castile, rue, senna leaves, linden, balm gentle, and mint.

Mexican Americans generally refer folk (culturally defined) illnesses to traditional healers or curers rather than to biomedical physicians, since the latter lack knowledge of such ailments and how to treat them. Both independent generalists and independent specialists function within the context of curanderismo. Curandera/os are independent generalists who treat a wide variety of physical and emotional problems. They possess *el don* (the gift of healing) that enables them to diagnose both naturalistic and supernaturalistic illnesses, including culture-bound syndromes such as *susto* (fright), *empacho* (the clogging of the stomach and upper intestinal tract from excessive food or the wrong kinds of food), *bilis* (jaundice-like condition resulting from anger or fear), *mal ojo* (evil eye), and *mal puesto* (witchcraft). Some curandera/os do not accept their gift until they have reached an advanced age, but others acknowledge it while still children (Madsen 1973:89). Based upon ethnographic research on Mexiquito—little Mexico—a barrio in New Lots (pseudonym), a small city in the lower Rio Grande Valley of south Texas, anthropologist Arthur Rubel reported that "each curandero [in the community] is closely identified with the spirit of a deceased healer" and that "curanderos are characterized by personal qualities of a deviant nature" (1966:180).

Trotter and Chavira (1981) delineate three levels of treatment employed by curandera/os: the material, the spiritual, and the mental. The material level entails the use of numerous herbs, patent medicines, common household items (e.g., eggs, lemons, garlic), and religious articles (e.g., holy water or oil, incense, perfumes), along with prayers, ritual sweepings, and cleansings. Curandera/os often prescribe foods and/or herbs to correct imbalances caused by exposure to cold air or by overeating of "hot" or "cold" foods. They also rely upon the use of magico-religious objects, such as votive candles and statues, and rituals in an effort to ward off hexes. At the spiritual level, the curandera/o is a medium who serves as a vessel for one of a wide array of spirits. Much of her effort aims at inspiring faith in her patients and sometimes even fear. At the mental level, the curandera channels mental energy from her or his mind directly to the afflicted part of the patient.

Some curandera/os have incorporated aspects of biomedicine into their treatment regimens. Based upon his study of curanderismo in Hildago County in the Lower Rio Grande Valley of southern Texas, Madsen reported the following concerning its interface with biomedicine:

> It is quite commonplace for *curanderos* to give their patients written prescriptions for herb medicines. These prescriptions are usually filled at drug stores across the border where the medicine is put in bottles or boxes with typed labels. A few *curanderos* give injections of vitamins or penicillin. Antibiotics can be purchased without prescription at drug stores in Mexico where druggists instruct the curer in the technique of giving hypodermic injections and tell him the standard dosages. (1973:91–92)

Some curandera/os equip their offices with biomedical instruments, such as stethoscopes and drug store medicines. Most, however, are reluctant to accept cases that they consider terminal and often refer such patients to a biomedical physician.

Romano-V. (1965) delineates the following hierarchical typology of Mexican American healers: (1) an elder daughter (14 years or older) who exhibits the gift of divine healing and treats family members; (2) the mother who also treats family members; (3) the grandmother who serves as an intermediary between other practitioners and family members; (4) the neighborhood curer (female or male) who renders services upon request; (5) the village or *barrio* healer who is referred to as a curandera or curandero and may draw her or his power from a particular saint; (6) the town or urban enclave healer (female or male) who caters to clients from different neighborhoods and may maintain a shrine for her or his patron saint; (7) the regional healer (male or female) who serves clients from several villages or cities; (8) the international healer (male or female) who treats clients from both the United States and Mexico; (9) the international folk saint who functioned as a highly exceptional healer while he or she was alive and is now regarded to be an intermediary with God but is not officially recognized by the Catholic church; and (10) the international, formal saint, exemplified by Our Lady of Guadalupe, the patron saint of Mexico. Don Pedrito Jarmillo and El Niño Fidencio are two curanderos who evolved into folk saints following their deaths. Don Pedrito, who practiced for 25 years, used herbalism, spiritualism, and hydrotherapy. He lived a life of self-imposed poverty in Texas and never married. Following Don Pedrito's death in 1907, his clients transformed him into a folk saint and his burial site into a shrine. Several curanderas and curanderos in Mexiquito adopted the names of Don Pedrito Jaramillo and El Fidencio, whom I discuss in greater detail in the following section on Mexican American spiritism (Rubel 1966:184).

Healers classified as independent specialists, the second major category within curanderismo, include *yerberos,* or herbalists; *sobadoras,* or masseuses/bone setters; *senoras,* or "wise women"; and *pateras,* or midwives. *Yerberos* are knowledgeable about hundreds of wild and domestic medicinal plants and home remedies. They tend not to diagnose but rather to prescribe medicines once a diagnosis has been made. *Yerberos* often operate out of a *yerberia* or *botanica*—a store that sells herbs as well as perfumes, oils, candles, and other mystical objects. *Sobadoras* treat muscle sprains and misaligned bones by massaging, rubbing, or kneading the affected part of the body (Anderson 1987). They are generally women who learned their skill from their mothers or grandmothers. *Senoras* are middle-aged or elderly women who read cards in order to inform their clients about their present, past, or future circumstances. They tend to treat members of their extended family or neighborhood. *Pateras* often stay at home expectant mothers from the time that their labor begins, administering massages, and providing hot teas. They are considered to be more patient than biomedical physicians but may refer clients to herbalists or biomedical clinics. Rubel (1966:181) reported that in 1955 the seven Mexiquito pateras registered with the Hidalgo County Health Unit delivered over twice as many Mexiquito infants as did M.D.s.

Some Mexican Americans patronize various types of heterodox practitioners, in addition to biomedical physicians. Residents of Sal si Puedes in San Jose reportedly sought treatment from chiropractors, homeopaths, and herbalists, many of whom advertised their services on Spanish-language radio or in Spanish-language newspapers (Clark 1970:211). Some residents were not aware of the difference between a chiropractor and a biomedical physician.

SPIRITISM OR ESPIRITISMO AMONG MEXICAN AMERICANS

Spiritists, or *espiritualistas,* who are usually women, function as mediums who are either leaders of or mediums in *templos,* or temples. Mexican and Mexican American spiritism, or *espiritismo,* is "mildly messianic, ecumenical, and overt" in that "spiritualists band together openly and actively attempt to attract new followers" (Kearney 1978:69). It is reportedly a growing religious movement in south Texas and other parts of the Southwest (Trotter and Chavira 1981:102–148). Whereas curanderismo has historically been associated with rural communities, spiritism, both in Mexico and the United States, tends to be associated with urban communities (Finkler 1985). Depending upon its size, a temple may have from one to 20 mediums. Some spiritists have established loose formal associations based upon friendship ties and geographical proximity. Espiritualistas tend to focus on psychosomatic and emotional disorders or problems of living.

Some spiritists undergo training at Mexican temples and display their certificates on their walls (Madsen 1973:91). Others obtain their certificates through correspondence courses administered by spiritist centers in Mexico. Spiritists often charge higher fees than do biomedical physicians. Consequently, they are frequently suspected of being charlatans. Nevertheless, their clients believe them to be particularly effective in treating bewitchment.

Macklin describes the practice of a spiritist medium, Juan Luis Martinez (pseudonym), who had organized a group of Mexican Americans in San Antonio and "follows the works of Trincado [an Argentine], whose 12 books are studied to develop such mediumistic abilities, including the power to heal" (1978:156). Martinez became an active medium in the Kardecist Spiritist Center in San Antonio by the early 1920s:

As Juan Luis's fame had spread, Trincado heard of him, wrote, and forwarded him his own books. Juan Luis came to consider Trincado—who prophesied that a utopian commune of the entire world, in which everyone would communicate in Spanish, could be expected by 1980—more progressive and "scientific" than Kardec. He was particularly attracted to the system's promise of equality and justice. . . . He launched, in 1931, the first regional Trincado spiritist school in the United States. (Macklin 1978:160)

Eventually, however, Juan Luis abandoned his struggle against the political economy in the United States and focused on a more traditional form of spiritism that sought the care of protecting spirits.

Some Mexican Americans are devotees of the spiritist folk saint El Niño Fidencio, who asserted that he had received his healing powers from the Heavenly Father. Fidencio, whose work received much attention from the Mexican media in the 1920s and 1930s, established a healing center in the tiny village of Espinazo in the state of Nuevo Leon (Zavaleta 1998). He reportedly performed surgery with a piece of glass from a broken bottle and kept a large number of bottles with tissue and tumors extracted from his patients. Fidencio told his followers that he would communicate with them through spirit mediums following his death, which occurred in 1938. The *Fidencista* movement has strongholds in major northern Mexican cities as well as missions in areas where Mexican migrant workers have settled, including parts of Texas, Indiana, Ohio, Michigan, Colorado, Washington, and Oregon (Zavaleta 1998:110). *Materias,* who were primarily women, established local missions. Three categories of devotees seek health care at Fidencista missions: a small inner circle of followers and assistants, a larger group consisting of regular attendees, and people seeking healing on an episodic basis. Devotees generally visit a Fidencista healer for help with a serious ailment or personal problem:

> Most of the regular members of a *Fidencista* temple make weekly appearances for simple blessings (*bendiciones*) and positive emotional reinforcement. Ritual sweepings, in which the healer uses a sweeping motion with herbs or special sacred objects, are used to rid the patient of "bad vibes." (Zavaleta 1998:112)

Zavaleta (1998:111) asserts that Fidencio is by far the most popular of the many Mexican and Mexican American folk saints and Catholic saints.

PUERTO RICAN ESPIRITISMO

Puerto Rican *espiritismo* is one of the many syncretic, trance-possession religions of the Caribbean. It blends Native American, African, and Roman Catholic beliefs and practices but draws primarily upon the writings of Allan Kardec. Although it was first in vogue in Puerto Rican high society, espiritismo spread to the urban poor and peasantry of the island. It evolved into a decentralized religious healing system with hundreds of *centros*, or temples, among working-class Puerto Ricans on the island and in the mainland United States (Garrison 1977a, 1977b). Puerto Rican espiritismo is now coming under the influence of Afro-Cuban santeria, incorporating Yoruban deities into its pantheon of spirits (Singer and Garcia 1989:160). It tends in large part to be an urban phenomenon and to cater, though not exclusively, to working-class Puerto Ricans.

Espiritismo focuses upon communication with the supernatural realm, which is occupied by numerous spirits. Spirits pass through a series of incarnations and can either protect the living or harass them by possessing them or by coming close enough to adversely affect them.

The politico-religious hierarchy of a centro consists of three status levels: the *Presidente*, or head, who serves as both the pastor and chief medium; the *mediunidads*, or assistant mediums, who help the head in exorcizing malevolent spirits and diagnosing clients' problems; and the herbalist (Harwood 1987:54–55). The head of a temple and his or her mediums attempt to achieve contact with the spirit realm in order to cure their clients. Mediums treat a broad range of problems, including *envidia* (envy), *brujeria* (sorcery), *mala influencia* (evil influence), *prueba* (test or trial), and *castigo* (punishment). Espiritualistas, or spiritists, are generally "wounded healers" who have rid themselves of some sort of affliction. These mediums feel their clients' ailments. They use spirit guides to identify the spirit causing the client's problem and manipulate religious symbols to overcome negative spiritual forces. Singer and Garcia note:

> Unlike biomedical practitioners, espiritas "view the client's symptoms as a gift or quality" . . . . Consequently, clients commonly are invited to undergo *desarralo* (spiritual development) to cultivate their innate *facultades* (spiritual abilities) and become mediums of the centro. Spiritual development involves the acquisition of new degrees of power by expanding one's relations with increasingly more potent spiritual beings. Mediums "win" a spirit by adhering to the centro's code of behavior, serving the spirit realm (e.g., by making offerings and saying prayers), and by exhibiting respect to the leading medium. (1989:160–61)

Mediums treat clients in both public and private settings. They also prescribe herbs, oils, candles, perfumes, and other religious paraphernalia, which may be purchased in stores called *botanicas*. Mediums and devotees use candles to dispel malevolent spirits from their homes, to petition the saints, or to perform sorcery. They perform ritual cleansings either by fumigation, which drives away evil spirits, or by washing with water or cologne, which attracts benevolent spirits.

Singer, along with two of his associates, conducted research on *Centro de Nuestro Padre Lazaro* (Center of Our Father Lazarus) in Hartford (Singer and

Borrero 1984; Singer and Garcia 1989). Marta de Jesus established the centro in May 1980 and served as its *madrina* (godmother). The centro was situated in a one-room storefront, which included the sanctuary, a small kitchen, a secluded healing area, and a small botanica that sold healing and protective articles such as herbs, cleansing baths, candles, incense, and statues of the Catholic saints and Yoruba gods. Marta had trained about two dozen spiritist mediums and attracted a large clientele in the Puerto Rican community. Singer and Garcia describe the clientele:

> Almost all mediums first come to the centro as clients seeking help for health, social, or spiritual problems. A recent study of fifty clients at the centro . . . found they report a high number (an average of ten per client) of stress-related symptoms, including frequent nausea, body pains, stomachaches, headaches, sleeplessness, loss of appetite, and dizziness and commonly feel anger, sadness, and depression. The most common presenting complaints of centro clients were found to be emotional problems (31 percent), family conflict (25 percent), general ill health (8 percent). Approximately half of the clients in the study feared that witchcraft or sorcery was contributing to the problems they were experiencing. Users of the centro apparently feel they benefit from the services offered to treat these conditions, because many become regular visitors and tell friends and relatives about the centro. (1989:177–78)

Koss-Chioino (1975) argues that espiritismo provides its adherents with control over lives. Spiritism labels the client's problem without stigmatizing him or her because the cause is attributed to external spirits. It also communicates to the client that others care about him or her and provides a therapeutic community, particularly for those who choose to become mediums.

SANTERIA AMONG CUBAN AMERICANS

Santeria is a syncretic Afro-Cuban religious healing system that draws upon Yoruba orisha worship, the Catholic cult of saints, and spiritism (González-Wippler 1982; Murphy 1992). The term *santeria* is derived from the Spanish term *santo* (saint). Many middle-class Cubans embraced espiritismo as a scientific and anti-Catholic belief system. When espiritismo filtered down to the lower classes and rural areas, it became intertwined with Catholicism. Afro-Cuban adherents came to associate the Yoruba gods or *orishas* with Catholic saints, thus laying the basis for santeria. As Brandon notes, santeria incorporates the "names and personalities of the African deities, divination procedures, ceremonial spirit possession and trance, liturgical music and musical instruments" (1990:121).

The earliest followers of santeria in the United States appear to have been priests, priestesses, and devotees who emigrated from Cuba in the mid-1940s

164

(Brandon 1990:120). Devotees of santeria came to the United States in increasing numbers after the Cuban revolution of 1959. It has taken root in several areas, particularly Florida, New York, New Jersey, and California (Sandoval 1979). In recent decades, santeria has been gaining popularity among African Americans, particularly in New York City (Curry 1997).

The relationship between orishas and the Catholic saints is complex. Male orishas may be represented by female and white saints or female orishas by male and white saints. Murphy (1988:121) asserts that the association between saint and *orisha* in santeria permits devotees to practice both European and African traditions. Orishas/saints, or santos, that concern themselves with health problems include Shango/St. Barbara, who deals with violent death; Babalu-Aye/St. Lazarus, who deals with illness in general; Basoso/St. Christopher, who deals with infections; and Ifa/St. Anthony, who deals with fertility (Spector 1996:292). Santeria is a highly syncretic and fluid religious healing system that elicits and accepts new elements, including some from Puerto Rican espiritismo. Indeed, santeria cult houses had become multiethnic as early as 1961, catering to both Cubans and Puerto Ricans. In time, santeria also attracted Panamanians, Colombians, Dominicans, African Americans, and even some European Americans, including those of Jewish extraction. *Santerismo* refers to the Puerto Rican variant of santeria which incorporates elements from espiritismo (Brandon 1993).

Practitioners of santeria worship in an *ile* (house) that may be situated in a building, a courtyard, or the home of a senior priest or priestess. The political-religious hierarchy of an ile consists of the head priest/priestess, the head medium, and the mediums. Initiation into the ile entails possession by an orisha who enthrones himself or herself on the head of the devotee. A santero (male medium) or santera (female medium) can use his or her magical powers to perform good or evil, including helping a client overcome negative influences, recover from an illness, secure employment, attract a lover or spouse, improve financial circumstances, or subdue or destroy rivals and enemies. According to Murphy,

> Perhaps the most important service offered by the ile is health care. *Santeras* and *santeros* are justly famous for their diagnostic skill and herbal treatments . . . priestesses and priests are expert in a vast pharmacopeia, and believers are quick to offer testimonies to the miraculous intervention of the *orishas* in effecting cures prescribed by *santeras* and *santeros.* (1994:87–88)

Santera/os use plants in healing rites, such as fumigation with cigar smoke, baths, house cleansings, and rites directed at the client's head (Brandon 1991). Santeria devotees believe in the power of consecrated objects such as stones containing the powers of the orishas. The stones are used to make protective necklaces and bracelets.

Santeria aims to provide its adherents with spiritual power to confront the realities of everyday life. It has created controversy and incurred the wrath of legal authorities in the United States because of its reliance upon the ritual sacrifice of animals such as chickens and goats. The U.S. Supreme Court overturned a series of ordinances prohibiting ritual animal sacrifices that the city of Hialeah, Florida, passed in the early 1990s. Justice Anthony Kennedy stated, "Although the practice of animal sacrifice may seem abhorrent to some, religious belief need not be acceptable, logical, consistent, or comprehensible to others in order to merit First Amendment protection" (quoted in Clark 1998:123).

Santeria reportedly has begun to move out of the inner city into the suburbs, where it has found new clients among African American, European American, and Asian American professional people (Clark 1998:129). Organizations such as the Caribbean Cultural Center in Manhattan and the Oni-Ochun Center in Oakland provide forums for the practice of a more public form of santeria.

THE CONTRADICTORY ROLE OF HISPANIC FOLK MEDICAL SYSTEMS

Like African American folk healers, Hispanic folk healers practice in both private and cultic settings. Hispanic folk medical systems provide partially holistic approaches to health problems in that they strongly emphasize the sociocultural, psychological, and spiritual factors contributing to illness (Sandoval 1979; Trotter and Chavira 1981; Harwood 1987). They tend to be congruent with Hispanic cultural and religious beliefs and generally allow for input from the patient's or client's family. Hispanic folk medical systems also serve as a counterbalance to the fragmentation of biomedical services for poor people, especially those who are undocumented workers. In many cases, folk healers provide Hispanics with a cheaper form of health care than do biomedical practitioners. Mexican American and Puerto Rican spiritist centers and Cuban American santeria houses provide familial religious and social meeting places for urban migrants and assist them in adjusting to urban life.

Curanderismo, Mexican American spiritism, Puerto Rican espiritismo, and santeria, like African American folk medicine, combine elements of protest and accommodation. They all provide an important source of cultural identity and pride for both practitioners and clients. Curandera/os, espiritualistas, and santera/os all function as folk psychiatrists in seeking to help their clients either transcend or at least adjust to difficulties in their lives (Kiev 1968; Garrison 1977a, 1977b; Harwood 1987). With respect to curanderismo, Trotter and Chavira argue that it combines self-reliance with cultural relevance and family systems and gives some Mexican Americans a sense of stability and continuity in the face of socially disrupting urban-technological change. It provides a linkage of past and future in a therapeutic system. (1981:174)

Hispanic folk healers encourage their clients to change at the individual level but do not generally encourage them to challenge existing political-economic arrangements in the larger society or to engage in social activism (Koss-Chioino 1975). Romano-V. (1965:1170) maintains that Don Pedrito was "more of a *renovator* than an *innovator*" and that he exemplified the "charisma of conservatism" because he encouraged his clients to maintain traditional Mexican American cultural patterns. Hispanic cultic centers tend to substitute high religious status for low social status, perhaps especially in the case of women. As Harwood observes, "spirit mediumship provides one of the few opportunities for a Puerto Rican woman to achieve formal leadership in a group composed of males and females" (1987:183). Some Hispanic folk healers, however, act as catalysts for social change. Marta, the *madrina* (godmother) of a centro in Hartford, played an active role in demonstrations after the hit-and-run death of a medium's child and protested the manner in which the city and police department handled the case against a prominent local attorney who was eventually convicted of the crime (Singer and Garcia 1989: 182). In addition to her public protests against poverty and discrimination,

> Marta regularly plays an advocacy role on behalf of her clients and fellow mediums. This commonly involves helping them to link up with community agencies or assisting them in receiving legal or financial aid. Through her contacts at the Hispanic Health Council [a community-based outreach and research center] and other Puerto Rican agencies, Marta is able to aid her clients in overcoming bureaucratic red tape and institutional racism that further complicates the lives of impoverished Puerto Rican families. (Singer and Garcia 1989:182–83)

Indeed, Marta regarded her social activism as an extension of her healing role in the centro.

EAST ASIAN AMERICAN FOLK MEDICAL SYSTEMS

As Koss-Chioino so aptly observes, "there is a great degree of variation between ethnomedical systems among Chinese, Japanese, Vietnamese, and tribal peoples such as the Hmong or Lao" (1995:154). Of these Asian medical systems, Chinese folk medicine has received the greatest attention.

Chinese folk medicine draws many of its concepts and practices from classical Chinese medicine. It attributes health problems to an excess of one thing or a deficiency of another thing, such as insufficient sleep, imbalanced diet in childhood, excessive work, or boredom, and characterizes foods, medicines, and diseases as either "hot" or "cold." The hot/cold dialectic may be related to changes in temperature from weather, bathing, or room conditions. *Chi*—a vitalistic energy—is believed to flow along various meridians in the body just as blood flows through the veins. Chinese folk medicine includes many home preventive health methods, including drinking cooling teas in hot weather, eating "cold" food in hot weather, drinking soups and eating dishes with herbs in cold weather, and drinking herbal teas.

Many Chinese American immigrants reside in or near Chinatowns in major cities, such as San Francisco, Oakland, Los Angeles, New York, Chicago, and Boston (Hessler et al. 1975). Chinese Americans often rely upon patent medicines from Taiwan, Hong Kong, and mainland China as well as Chinese doctors who diagnose minor problems from the patient's appearance, make pulse diagnoses, perform acupuncture, prescribe herbs, administer moxibustion, and set bones. Chinese doctors often practice in the back rooms of gift shops in Chinatowns and have learned their practice through apprenticeships. As noted previously, acupuncture and other therapeutic techniques associated with Chinese medicine have become increasingly popular among European Americans, in large part under the rubric of the holistic health movement (see Barnes 1998). According to Hare, "one of the most striking aspects of the incorporation of Chinese medical systems into Western health care is the degree to which there is a mixing of classical Chinese, other scholarly or professional East Asian, and modern Chinese medical thought, with a variety of folk paradigms from East Asia and the many ethnic streams of the Western locale in which the new 'Oriental' medicine is now being practiced" (1993: 38).

Japanese American folk medicine is based in part on Chinese medicine as well as on forms of religious healing within the Buddhist and Shinto traditions, but unfortunately it has received little attention from social scientists. One study has been conducted by James V. Spickard (1991), who investigated the San Francisco mission of Sekai Kyusek-kyo (Church of World Messianity), a syncretic healing sect that emerged as one of the 700 or so "new religions" established in Japan in the nineteenth and twentieth centuries. Mokichi Okada founded World Messianity after he had been visited by the Buddhist goddess of Mercy, Kannon. He received a series of revelations that provided guidelines for humans to help bring about a New Age of truth, beauty, and an earthly paradise. Okada taught that believers can serve as harbingers of the New Age who spread a Divine Light to others by wearing "an *ohikari* ('sacred focal point') around their necks, which allows them to channel *johrei*"—a spiritual energy which replaces illness and misery with genuine health and happiness and purifies the world and the soul (Spickard 1991:140).

When Spickard conducted fieldwork on World Messianity in the mid-1970s, he found that

> the core of the church—over half of the membership—was made up of middle-aged Nisei (second generation) Japanese-Americans. They were predominantly middle-class or upper working-class; many were successful landscapers and truck farmers (or their wives), or the owners of small businesses—traditional occupations for first and second generation Japanese in California. Their median age was 45–50; both women and men attended church functions, though women were more active. (1991:143)

Most middle-aged Japanese Americans attended the mission because they believed johrei brought them material prosperity and health; they tended to be uninterested in the coming of a New Age. "Older white" members, who made up about 25 to 30 percent of the congregation, had joined World Messianity after their children had grown up. Most had dabbled in other esoteric sects, such as Spiritualism, Rosicrucianism, and Anthroposophy. They had a higher regard for the ancient wisdom and spirituality of Japan than did the Japanese American members. In contrast to their Japanese American age-set counterparts, the "older white" members were more interested in the spiritual than in the physical benefits of johrei. Finally, "younger white" members, most of whom identified with the counterculture movement, tended to stress the belief in a New Age. Many of the "older whites" and "younger whites" left the sect after the Mother Church in Japan sent teams of ministers to re-orient the membership. Although most middle-aged Japanese attended re-dedication classes, "these members continued to used *johrei* primarily for personal benefits—despite warnings against doing so" (Spickard 1991:148).

Some research has been conducted on other East Asian immigrant groups. Folk medicine among Hmong refugees in the United States has received a modest amount of scholarly attention (Muecke 1983; O'Connor 1995:80–108). Capps (1994) identified four female herbalists in her ethnographic study of the medical culture of the Hmong in Kansas City, Kansas. She reported that the Kansas City Hmong disregarded some traditional Hmong medical beliefs such as soul loss and spirit illness. Instead, they adapted their indigenous beliefs to Protestantism by expressing concerns about illness in group prayers. The Kansas City Hmong, however, continued to believe in fright illness—a condition that is treated either by massage or prayer rather than the traditional shamanistic soul-calling ritual. Hmong medical culture also includes elements of Chinese medicine, including adherence to the humoral concept that excessive emotion can cause illness, and the practice of needling as a means of releasing bad blood or air. Although biomedicine plays a minor role in Hmong beliefs about health and illness, Hmong refugees rely upon it for prenatal care, immunization, and the treatment of certain diseases, such as hypertension and diabetes.

NATIVE AMERICAN HEALING SYSTEMS

In a sense, there are as many Native American healing systems as there are Native American ethnic groups in the United States. Native American healing systems are intricately intertwined with Native American religions. Despite their diversity, they share a view of humans as an integral part of nature and consider the restoration of spiritual power as central for attaining health (Lyon 1996:xiii). Traditional Native American healing systems tend to focus upon psychological, rheumatic, urinary, and gastro-intestinal ailments as well as rashes, fractures, wounds, and eye irritations (the latter largely a result of living in smoky dwellings). At least in the past, they did not deal with epidemic diseases, cancer, and cardiovascular complications because these did not exist or rarely occurred. Native American medicine became popular on the North American frontier and had a strong impact upon European American and African American folk medicine. Anthropologist Daniel E. Moerman asserts that "native Americans were acute observers of nature, competent botanists, superb psychiatrists, and excellent physicians" (1981:12). European Americans obtained from Native Americans a cure for scurvy, methods of oral contraception, and over 200 medicinal substances listed in the *U.S. Pharmacopeia.*

Native American healing systems are both empirical and spiritual in their approaches to restoring imbalances between individuals and their sociocultural environments. They tend to rely upon three basic techniques: (1) herbs and drugs; (2) mechanical interventions, such as sweat baths, soaking in mineral baths, isolation of sick persons, and surgery; and (3) contact with the spirit realm. Like folk medical systems in general, they generally emphasize the attainment of harmony in social relations.

Illness is generally thought to result from sorcery (a common belief among some southwestern groups such as the Zuni, Navajo, and Yaqui), taboo violation, the intrusion of a foreign object or spirit, or soul loss (a common belief among the Inuit). Illnesses may manifest themselves in one of two ways: a spirit or disease object intrudes into the body or mind, or a spirit steals the victim's soul or power. In the former case, the shaman or healer attempts to frighten the intrusive agent away or to remove it from the body by sucking, fanning, or drawing it out. In the latter case, the healer goes into a trance in which his or her soul attempts to retrieve the runaway or stolen soul.

170

Plains Indian medicine men conduct sweat lodge ceremonies for a small number of males in small dome-shaped lodges constructed of saplings, hides, and blankets (Powers 1989:21). The medicine man creates a great rush of hot air by sprinkling water over heated stones. The participants sing and petition special favors from the spirits who enter the lodge, and they also pray for the general welfare of their tribe. Whereas in the past the sweat lodge ceremony was conducted as a preparation for battle, a horse-raiding venture, a vision quest, or the Sun Dance, today it serves as a means of purifying individuals both physically and spiritually. The Lakota of the Pine Ridge Reservation in South Dakota resort to sweating as a means of overcoming physical ailments (including AIDS), achieving tranquility, renewing friendships, and overcoming personal problems, including drug addiction and alcoholism (Bucko 1998). According to Bucko, "in the contemporary sweat lodge, different people attribute healing to a variety of sources: intercession of the spirits with God, the power and recommendations of the spirits themselves, the power of Tunkashila or Wakan Tanka, the power of the rocks (themselves seen as spirits or grandfathers) or the strea, or the physical effects of the lodge itself." The Oglala Lakota regard social solidarity as more important than religious orthodoxy in achieving a cure.

Many Native American groups or tribes characteristically had or have a number of different types of healers. Hultkrantz (1992:18) delineates three types of Native American healers: the herbalist, the "ordinary" medicine man or woman, and the shaman. The herbalist deals with simple wounds, aches, and musculoskeletal problems and relies upon medicinal plants, magico-religious rituals, and purifying substances such as incense and emetics. Kindscher (1992) identified 172 medicinal plants that the Indians living on the prairies employed. The "ordinary" medicine man or woman uses magico-religious rituals in his or her healing activities. The shamans are medicine men or women of a special sort who make contact with the supernatural realm on behalf of the patient by falling into a deep trance or ecstasy. Healers tend to function as solo practitioners, often having received a call to cure from the spirits, and generally conduct healing rituals as group events that are attended by kinfolk and other community members. Plains Indian medicine people were compensated in the past with horses, buffalo robes, or blankets but now receive food or money as payment.

Healers or shamans in many North American Indian tribes belong to medicine societies. In some tribes, healers are initiated into medicine societies through a series of rituals. The Iroquois have eight medicine societies: (1) the Society of Medicine Men, who receive healing power after offering a feast in honor of a guardian animal spirit; (2) the Company of Mystic Animals (e.g., the Buffalo, Otter, Bear, and Eagle societies), whose shamans receive curing powers from guardian animal spirits; (3) the Little Water Medicine

171

Society, which was originally associated with the healing of war wounds; (4) the Little People Society, which fosters rapport between its members and the *jo-ga-ob* ("little people"), elf-like spirits who assist humans in various ways; (5) the False Face Society, whose members obtain healing power by wearing wooden masks representing different spirits; (6) the Husk Faces Society, whose members implore spirits who will ensure successful farming; (7) the *Towii'sas* Society, consisting of women who honor corn, beans, and squash; and (8) the *Ohgiwe* Society, which conducts ceremonies for people who have been dreaming of ghosts (St. John 1989:135–36).

The Chippewa or Ojibwa of the western Great Lakes region had a hierarchy that included four categories of healers: (1) "the priests of the *Midewiwin*, or medicine society, to which membership was gained by initiation and payment of gifts;" (2) the *Wabenos*, or "dawn men," who provided hunting medicine, love powder, and other medicinal substances; (3) the *"Jessakid*, seers and prophets, revealers of hidden truths, possessors of a gift of clairvoyance received from the thunder god;" and (4) *Masshki-kike-winini*, or herbalists (Vogel 1970:22). Different Chippewa healers often used different medicinal plants and may have used different names for the same plant (Densmore 1974: 323).

Shamans and medicine men in Plains Indian societies carried around their necks or waists medicine bags that held sacred stones, shells, herbs, and other objects (Null 1998:64–66). The bags were made from the hide of an animal such as a deer or bear and were believed to provide protection from harm. In the past, Cheyenne healers specialized; some of them treated gunshot wounds, some provided war medicines, and some provided the power to fly or run fast (Moore 1996:237–38). Since only a few traditional Cheyenne doctors exist today, they generally use different medicines derived from different sources.

Hultkrantz asserts that traditional Native American healing practices today are "sometimes hidden to the outsider, much more so than in earlier days — a general consequence of Native discontent with anthropological observers. Yet in some cases Native Americans have pursued an aggressive medical program, challenging the supremacy of white medicine" (1992:3).

The remainder of this section focuses on four of the many Native American healing systems: Comanche eagle doctoring, Navajo medicine, Lumbee herbal medicine, and peyotism. The first three constitute examples of traditional healing systems and the latter, particularly as exemplified in the Native American Church, is an example of a more recent development in Native American healing.

COMANCHE EAGLE DOCTORING

David E. Jones (1972) provides a detailed ethnographic account of the healing endeavors of Sanapia (1895–1968), a Comanche eagle doctor. After completing seven years of formal education at the Cache Creek Mission School in southern Oklahoma, Sanapia embarked, at the age of 14, upon a four-year apprenticeship to become a healer under the tutelage of her mother and her mother's older brother, both of whom were eagle doctors. In the first phase of her training, Sanapia learned how to identify certain medicinal plants in the field and how to prepare and administer them. She next learned how to diagnose and treat various illnesses. Finally, Sanapia learned about the rules of conduct associated with healing. As a Comanche medicine woman, she functioned as a medium who possessed *paha*, or the supernatural power through which Medicine operates. In later life, Sanapia was honored, following four days and nights of seclusion and meditation, with a visitation by the eagle, her guardian spirit. She also made contact with the supernatural realm by consuming peyote at peyote ceremonies that she regularly attended.

Sanapia carried several types of botanical and nonbotanical medicines in a leather case and wrapped each medicine in a cloth. She used a bundle of four crow feathers while healing in order to ward off ghosts and fanned patients ceremonially with an eagle feather. She used a sucking horn when sucking illness from the bodies of her patients, thereby preventing her from coming into direct contact with an infectious wound. Sanapia specialized in the treatment of ghost sickness—a form of partial facial paralysis (see Henderson and Adour 1981)—and witch sickness.

Although Sanapia drew heavily upon traditional Comanche medicine, she also incorporated elements of Christianity and peyotism. Before beginning treatment, she held the Bible in both hands while praying for power. In her final years, Sanapia came to feel as though she were a "slightly outmoded necessity in Comanche society" and the purveyor of a dying tradition (Jones 1972:45). She was a "native psychiatrist" who treated the "individual rather than a specific static human affliction" (Jones 1972:104). As Jones notes, "this dynamic flexibility has enabled Comanche eagle doctors to exist long after the other varieties of Comanche doctors have had their function usurped by white doctors during the ongoing process of acculturation" (1972:104).

NAVAJO MEDICINE

Navajo religion adopted many aspects of Pueblo religion; it is predominantly "health-oriented" and seeks to establish a harmonious relationship between humans, nature, and the supernatural realm (Levy 1983:118). Indeed, Navajo religion consists in large part of a set of some 36 healing ceremonies (often

173

referred to as "sings" or "chants"), each lasting from one to nine days and nights. The Navajo of the American Southwest attribute disease to various causes, including sorcery, intruding spirits, and inappropriate actions, which are punished by the Holy People.

The hierarchy of healers in Navajo medicine includes the hand trembler, who diagnoses illnesses; the singer; the herbalist; and the bonesetter. The hand trembler does not attempt to cure illnesses but rather to ascertain their source:

> Through different techniques he solves the problem. He sits outside the sick man's or woman's hogan, listening to the winds, the animals, and the spirits. He also guides his hand feelingly over the body of the patient, and when he knows the nature of the disease his hand starts trembling. This capacity is a gift from a poisonous lizard, the so-called Gila Monster known to shake its forelegs. (Hultkrantz 1992:133–34)

The hand trembler prescribes the chant that needs to be followed in order to cure the illness. The singer performs what Topper (1987:223–25) terms "prophylactic" psychotherapeutic ceremonies, such as protection prayers for individuals who are or may become out of balance with the universe and the Blessing Way. Singers are generally males, although a few women have functioned in this capacity. In his hogan, the singer creates a mythic sandpainting and then destroys it with his feet as a symbolic enactment of the restoration of harmony in both the patient and his or her social network. A Navajo sing blends together many elements—songs, prayers, sandpaintings, and ritualistic items such as the medicine bundle, prayer-sticks, precious stones, tobacco, water collected from sacred places, or a tiny piece of cotton string. Sandpaintings exemplify the centrality of symbols to Navajo healing, since they must carefully follow traditional patterns that "recall significant episodes of mythical drama":

> The patient in his or her plight is identified with the cultural hero who constructed a similar disease or plight in the same way the patient did. . . . From the myth the patient learns that his or her plight and illness is not new, and that both its cause and treatment are known. To be cured, all the patient has to do is to repeat what has been done before. It has to be done sincerely, however, and this sincerity is expressed in concentration and dedication. The sandpainting depicts the desired order of things, and places the patient in this beautiful and ordered world. The patient thus becomes completely identified with the powerful and curing agents of the universe. (Witherspoon 1977:167–68)

The Holy Way and Evil Way chants are used primarily for mental disorders and the Life Way chants for physical ailments. Ultimately, healing is directed toward restoring harmony in the patient's life and in the members of his or her social network present at the chant.

174

In 1970, in response to the gradual decline of traditional Navajo healers, the National Institute of Mental Health created the Navajo Healing Arts Training Program—a project that reportedly trained some 90 individuals (Levy 1983:120). The Navajo Medicine Men's Association (est. 1979) attracted only a few singers and found its greatest appeal among diviners, herbalists, and peyote road chiefs. Topper maintains that the "traditional Navajo medicine man is . . . best described as a man of at least middle age who has earned a reputation in this community for knowledge, domestic stability, dependability and economic success" (1987:219). According to Kaplan and Johnson a substantial portion of the singers are "of the solid core of Navaho society" and the "highly successful singer may eventually become a comparatively wealthy man" (1964:222).

LUMBEE HERBAL MEDICINE

Edward M. Croon, Jr. (1992), an ethnobotanist, conducted a study of herbal medicine among the Lumbee Indians of Robeson County, North Carolina. The Lumbee reportedly are the largest Native American group east of the Mississippi River, but their identity as "Indians" has been contested by both the federal government and other Indian groups. The Lumbee appear to be a tri-hybrid group of Indian, European American, and African American ancestry. Croon asserts that although their lifestyle closely resembles that of white working-class Southerners, Lumbee folk medicine constitutes an important marker of their ethnic identity:

> One major body of lore linking the Lumbee to other Native Americans in the region is that concerning the use of herbal remedies to treat illness. Like many Indian groups in the United States, the Lumbee have a medical system that combines the use of herbal remedies with the magical treatment of disease by conjurers. Traditional Lumbee conjurers worked spells to cure the sick, predict the future, and influence the course of interpersonal events. While most Lumbee today consult physicians and utilize scientific medicine on a regular basis, many still rely on the use of herbal remedies to both prevent disease and treat routine conditions. (1992:140)

Based upon interviews in 1977–78 with 25 Lumbee herbalists (12 men and 13 women) over the age of 60, Croon identified 87 species that his subjects used as medicinal plants. Of these, 75 percent were local, readily available plants, 8 percent were cultivated plants, and 17 percent were rare in the wild or were obtained from outside Robeson County. Lumbee herbalists generally harvest plants immediately prior to processing them into teas, salves, and ointments. They sometimes prescribe teas brewed from several plants. The Lumbee use medicinal plants for diverse ailments, including circulatory, pulmonary, and kidney complications, skin rashes, insect and snake bites, and constipation, and even as tonics to stimulate hair growth. They utilize *Ambrosia* to treat diabetes, *Chimaphila* to treat neuritis, *Elaphantopus* to treat pneumonia, *Helenium* to treat allergies, asthma, and diabetes, *Rhus* to treat pellagra, and *Sisyrinchium* to treat colds, influenza, and pneumonia. Croon maintains that "Lumbee plant remedies should be seen as the foundation of a popular medical system whose pharmaceutical agents remain largely unproven by scientific studies" (1992:152).

PEYOTISM

Peyotism is a pan-Indian religious healing system that was imported from Mexico in the late nineteenth century and mixes elements of traditional Indian cultures, especially those of the Great Plains, with Christianity. Peyotists regard peyote—a cactus button containing the hallucinogenic agent mescaline—as a God-given sacramental element that helps them cope with the vagaries of life. The peyote plant is found in Mexico and Texas. Peyotism was first legally recognized in the institutionalized form of the Native American Church in Oklahoma in 1918 and has received similar recognition in other states. The majority of peyotists belong to southern Plains tribes, but members of other tribes, including the Navajo, belong to the sect.

Peyote meetings are conducted for special purposes such as curing ceremonies, birthday celebrations, funerals, memorial services, or when people leave an Indian community to travel long distances or return from military service. The peyote ritual is performed during an all-night meeting which includes praying, meditating, singing, drumming, and the consumption of peyote. A "roadman" or "roadchief," assisted by a drum chief and a fireman, leads the ceremony and gives attention to the illnesses of attendees or their relatives or friends by including them in prayers. Peyote meetings can be called whenever an individual experiences a social, spiritual or health need. Koss-Chioino maintains that peyotism engenders therapeutic effects in two ways:

> first, through a curing ceremony in which members of the church are treated for specific problems, often physical but also psychosocial (e.g. alcoholism) or emotional in nature. One traditional technique used is that of sucking out the evil spirit in the patient while other members sing and pray. Confession of sins at the ceremony is also employed. Second, the ceremony itself includes a number of therapeutic aspects: Conversion occurs by taking peyote or having a revelation, then being purged of sins through the physical purging brought on by the drug. Strong emotions in all participants are facilitated by the ceremony, accompanied by clear moral injunctions regarding abstinence from alcohol, marital fidelity, restraint from vengeance and fighting, and so on. (1995:157)

Peyotism is not a monolithic religious healing system but rather exhibits considerable diversity from one tribe to another as well as variation within a specific tribe. Two variations of peyotism, for example, had developed in Oklahoma by 1885 (Wiedman 1990). The Kiowa, Comanche, and Apache developed the Little Moon ritual, while the Delaware-Caddo developed the more elaborate Big Moon ritual that incorporated additional ritual roles, material items, and symbolism. Over time, the Big Moon ritual ceased among the Quapaw, Delaware, and other Oklahoma tribes, and by 1970 it was practiced only by the Osage. The Little Moon ritual replaced the Big Moon ritual among the Delaware. Wiedman contends that "many factors affected Big Moon Peyotism's decline in Northeast Oklahoma, including Delaware intermarriage with Euroamericans, acculturation to urban life, and acceptance of Western medical care" (1990:379). Moore (1996:251) asserts that the Cheyenne of Oklahoma and Montana regard the Native American Church as a "medicine lodge," which people visit primarily in order to overcome alcoholism, rather than as a "church" per se.

THE CONTRADICTORY ROLES OF CONTEMPORARY NAVAJO RELIGIOUS HEALING AND PAN-TRIBAL PEYOTISM

Both contemporary Navajo religious healing and peyotism as a pan-tribal movement constitute significant alternatives to biomedicine, which has become widespread among Native Americans especially in the form that is delivered by the Indian Health Service. They are both also important mechanisms for furthering and reinforcing Indian cultural identity. Topper contends that the Navajo medicine man serves as a "source of cultural and emotional stability and continuity" (1987:244), and Wiedman maintains that peyotism "functions as a health care delivery system by addressing health needs which are not fully met by the biomedical approach of orthodox, or other traditional healing systems" (1990:384).

Despite the presence of counterhegemonic elements in Navajo religious healing and peyotism, both, like so many other folk medical systems, ultimately tend to function as coping mechanisms that encourage their clients to adjust to the realities of European American–dominated society. Indeed, successful Navajo medicine men are petit bourgeois entrepreneurs who, unlike most of their impoverished Navajo neighbors, may own large numbers of livestock and enjoy the material amenities of American capitalism. While they are not officially political leaders, they frequently ally themselves with tribal leaders and may "influence and even control large blocks of votes in tribal elections" (Topper 1987:220). Navajo medicine men have often unwittingly become allies with Navajo tribal leaders who have made accommodations with the corporations that, with the assistance of the federal government, expropriate valuable energy resources from Navajo lands and, in some instances, have exposed Navajo miners and other reservation dwellers to the health hazards of radioactive waste materials (Churchill and LaDuke 1985).

Peyotism developed as an introversionist revitalization movement that spread after the demise of the Ghost Dance religion, which came to a sudden end with the massacre at Wounded Knee at the Pine Ridge Reservation in 1890. The Ghost Dance religion challenged the encroaching European American frontier political economy; peyotism, by contrast, called for personal transformation rather than social structural transformation. Although peyotism historically has functioned as a significant mechanism for overcoming alcoholism, its effectiveness has been limited and often temporary. In his case study of the role of peyotism in curbing heavy drinking among the Nebraska Winnebago, Hill observes:

> Individuals who tried Peyotism, but continued to believe that heavy drinking was acceptable behavior, or individuals who wished to change their drinking behavior, but remained with relatives and friends who did not support the new standards and behavior, might well continue to drink. Those who aspired to become successful farmers, but who were unable to acquire sufficient land due to the fractionalization of their allotments among many heirs, or who did not have sufficient funds to purchase draft teams or mechanized farming equipment, could become discouraged and turn to alcohol for consolation. And indeed, as the Winnebago moved further into the 20th century, the influence of Peyotism on the tribe lessened and heavy drinking again increased, even among those who claimed to be Peyotists. (1990:260)

Both traditional Navajo medicine and pan-tribal peyotism function as significant coping mechanisms for their adherents. While both contain subtle counterhegemonic elements, such as an effort to maintain Native American identity, neither offers a serious challenge to biomedical domination.

As is the case in Anglo-American religious healing systems such as Spiritualism, Christian Science, and Pentecostalism, folk medical systems among European Americans, African Americans, Haitian Americans, Hispanic Americans, Asian Americans, and Native Americans tend to merge religion and medicine—a pattern that also occurs in indigenous or tribal healing systems. Whereas Anglo-American religious healing systems tend to cut across socioeconomic lines, folk medical systems tend to cater by and large to working-class people. Finally, women often function as folk healers.

9

Conclusion

Shortly following the turn of the twentieth century, American medicine evolved from a relatively pluralistic system into a dominative one in which biomedicine became preeminent. Biomedicine claimed scientific superiority and established clear hegemony over alternative medicine as a result of financial backing first from corporate-sponsored foundations and later from the federal government for its research and educational institutions. The American dominative medical system consists of several levels that tend to reflect class, racial/ethnic, and gender relations in the larger society. In order of prestige, these include: (1) biomedicine; (2) osteopathic medicine; (3) professionalized heterodox medical systems (chiropractic, naturopathy, and acupuncture); (4) partially professionalized heterodox medical systems (e.g., homeopathy, herbalism, bodywork, and hypnotherapy); (5) Anglo-American religious healing systems (e.g., Spiritualism, Christian Science, Pentecostalism, Scientology); and (6) folk medical systems (e.g., southern Appalachian herbal medicine, African American folk medicine, *vodun, curanderismo, espiritismo, santeria,* East Asian folk medicines, and Native American healing traditions).

As we have seen, despite the biomedical establishment's attempts to restrict the practice of alternative healers, a number of heterodox medical systems continue to thrive in both rural and urban areas in the United States, and indeed throughout the world. Osteopathic physicians have obtained full practice rights, and some other practitioners—chiropractors, naturopaths, and acupuncturists—have obtained limited practice rights. Although women, minorities, and members of lower social classes often use alternative medical systems as a way to challenge the hegemony of biomedicine, ultimately the persistence of these systems is dependent on the willingness of strategic elites to permit their existence. Folk healing systems are more generally the domain of the common people, but, unfortunately, according to Elling, "traditional medicine has been used to obfuscate and confuse native peoples and working classes" (1981:97). Many heterodox and folk medical practitioners are inter-

179

ested in acquiring new skills and in using certain biomedical-like treatments or technologies in their own work, a process by which they often inadvertently adopt the reductionist perspective of biomedicine. In essence, even though biomedicine and alternative medical systems are antagonistic, they exhibit a great deal of overlap and even fusion.

Because of the bureaucratic dimensions of biomedicine and the frequent iatrogenic situations or mishaps that occur in the course of biomedical treatment, various alternative systems under the umbrella of the holistic health movement have either made a comeback or been developed in North America, western Europe, and other parts of the world in the last few decades. This eclectic movement, which incorporates elements from Asian medical systems, the human potential movement, New Ageism, as well as earlier Western heterodox medical systems, has begun to attract the attention of some biomedical practitioners.

THE GROWING INTEREST OF BIOMEDICAL PHYSICIANS AND NURSES IN HOLISTIC MEDICINE

The growing interest and/or concern of biomedical practitioners in holistic health is exemplified by the fact that the *Journal of the American Medical Association* devoted its November 11, 1998, issue to "alternative medicine." The holistic health movement, however, faces the danger of being co-opted by biomedicine as a growing number of biomedical physicians are turning to heterodox treatment regimens in response to the rejection of conventional biomedicine by their patients (Goldstein et al. 1987). As Alster so astutely observes,

> The physicians themselves . . . have reason to fear losing their "own piece of the action." In response to this possibility, some of them have adopted an "If you can't beat 'em, join 'em" approach, adopting holistic practices in varying degrees. The frequent calls for "integration" of holistic and traditional practices may serve the purpose of preserving the hegemony of medicine by co-opting the most attractive components of holism. (1989:163)

In a similar vein, James S. Gordon, a holistic M.D. and an enthusiast of holistic health centers, warns that there is a danger that they "will continue to be primarily a luxury for the wealthy, that their doctrine of self-help and individual responsibility will be perverted to public neglect" (1984:246).

Since the 1970s, more and more biomedical physicians have turned their attention to the holistic health movement. Some 220 physicians established the American Holistic Medical Association (AHMA) in 1978 (Pizer 1982: 115). Clyde Norman Shealy, founder of the Pain Rehabilitation Center in

La Crosse, Wisconsin, was elected as the first president. In the early 1990s the organization's membership reportedly included 521 physicians and 17 other health care providers (Fugh-Berman 1993:241). In 1980, the AHMA established the American Holistic Medical Foundation, an open-membership organization for people interested in holistic health care. Some physicians use other terms besides "holism" for alternative approaches. According to Collinge, "practitioners who were originally trained in other traditions [including biomedicine] and now use naturopathic principles often describe their work as 'natural' medicine rather than 'naturopathic' medicine" (1996:128). Many holistic M.D.s and D.O.s refer to their approach as "integrative medicine."

Andrew Weil, a Harvard-trained family physician at the University of Arizona, has become the most prominent holistic M.D. in the United States and probably the world. Several of his books have become best-sellers—*The Natural Mind* (1972), *Health and Healing* (1983), *Natural Health, Natural Medicine: A Comprehensive Manual for Wellness and Self Care* (1990), and *Spontaneous Healing* (1995)—and he has produced a videotape titled *Spontaneous Healing*. Although he contends that alternative medicine is a "mixed bag" in terms of its efficacy, he advocates the integration of "standard medicine" and "alternative medicine." Weil recently became the editor-in-chief of *Integrative Medicine: Integrating Conventional & Alternative Medicine*, a quarterly journal devoted to "the best concepts and techniques of a wide variety of health care practices."

Another well-known holistic M.D. is Deepak Chopra, author of *Perfect Health: The Complete Mind-Body Guide* (1990) and several other popular health books, who has introduced the American public to Ayurvedic medicine. James S. Gordon, another Harvard-trained physician, wrote *Holistic Medicine* (1988) and *Manifesto for a New Medicine: Your Guide to Healing Partnerships and the Wise Use of Alternative Therapies* (1996). Gordon is a clinical professor in the department of psychiatry and family medicine at Georgetown University and director of the Center for Mind-Body Medicine in Washington, D.C., and served as chairperson of the Program Advisory Council of the Office of Alternative Medicine.

The first teaching program in alternative medicine at an American biomedical institution was established in the 1970s at Montefiore Medical Center in the Bronx (Abrams 1994:99). Several medical schools, including those at Harvard, Tufts, Georgetown, and the University of Louisville, and some hospitals have incorporated alternative therapies into their programs of study and health services (Barash 1992). The Stress Reduction Center at the University of Massachusetts–Worcester Medical School teaches Buddhist meditation and yoga to patients. The Program in Integrative Medicine at the University of Arizona, directed by Andrew Weil, opened an integrative medicine clinic in 1997 (Ostgarden 1997:5). The American Association of Public Health has established a special primary interest group (SPIG) on alternative medicine whose members are both health practitioners and researchers (Gesler and Gordon 1998:9).

Only two studies to date, both directed by sociologist Michael S. Goldstein, have systematically attempted to provide a social profile of holistic physicians. In the first, Goldstein et al. (1985) interviewed 30 members of Physicians in Transition (PIT), a support group for holistically oriented physicians which was established at the Center for the Healing Arts in Los Angeles in 1975. For the most part, these physicians, who came from a diversity of specialities and practices, were actively involved in practicing biomedicine and "identified themselves as 'holistic' not on the basis of using specific nonmainstream techniques but, rather, on the basis of the overall context in which such techniques were used" (Goldstein et al. 1985:321). All of the physicians studied expressed dissatisfaction and/or disillusionment with biomedicine. Areas of dissatisfaction included limitations in the treatment of chronic diseases, iatrogenic dimensions, and restricted approach to the physician-patient relationship. Seven PIT members were influenced by personal experiences with psychotherapy, encounter groups, or other personal growth situations (Goldstein et al. 1985:329). Almost half the group (14) reported that personal rather than professional experience with illness had played some significant part in their involvement with holistic medicine:

> In 8 cases these illnesses had been their own, and in the remainder illness afflicted either spouses, lovers, or parents, with recovery occurring in most cases (10 of 14). . . . Ironically, in only 2 of the cases was contact with a physician or other healer identified as having influenced thinking about medicine, holism, or healing. (Goldstein et al. 1985:330–31)

As might be expected, half of the interviewees experienced hostility from their biomedical colleagues. Nevertheless, two-thirds of them maintained that their status as holistic M.D.s had not disrupted their personal lives.

In a second study, Goldstein and his colleagues compared 340 members of the American Holistic Medical Association with 142 family practice physicians (FPs) in California (Goldstein et al. 1987, 1988). Although the groups were similar in age, sex, and social class origin, there were significant differences among them:

> AMHAs are significantly less likely than FPs to have been raised in metropolitan environments and to have attended an American medical school; roughly equal proportions graduated from foreign medical schools (9.9% versus 5.1% of the FPs) and from American osteopathic medical schools (10.2% versus 2.2% of the FPs). Thus foreign medical graduates, who constitute about one-fifth of all physicians in the United States, are underrepresented among both groups, while

osteopaths, who make up 3.9 percent of all U.S. physicians, are underrepresented among the FPs and overrepresented among AMHAs. (Goldstein et al. 1987:107)

Whereas 59.8 percent of the AMHAs regarded religion and/or spirituality as a "very important" dimensions of their lives, only 17.6 percent of the FPs did so (Goldstein et al. 1987: 110). AMHAs also participated more often in encounter groups or organized "personal growth experiences" than did FPs. Two-fifths (40.5 percent) of the AMHAs described their practices as "holistic," in contrast to 3.6 percent of the FPs (Goldstein et al. 1988:856).

Sociologist June S. Lowenberg (1989) conducted an in-depth ethnography of the "Mar Vista Clinic," a holistic health center emphasizing preventive family practice. The clinic was located in a major California city and did not refer to itself as "holistic," despite the fact that its practitioners identified themselves with the holistic health movement. The clinic's founder was also a founding member of both the AHMA and the Association of Holistic Health and held a master's degree in acupuncture. Mar Vista Clinic was served by an interdisciplinary team consisting of two family physicians, two registered nurses, two clinical psychologists, and two body workers. Patients at the clinic ranged from those who practiced holistic health as a lifestyle to those who were referred to the clinic. The vast majority of its patients were middle to upper middle class, and 60 percent were female. "Most clients had fairly high educational levels, and were extremely sophisticated consumers in medical matters" (Lowenberg 1989:100). Mar Vista Clinic's services included family practice medicine, traditional acupuncture, nutritional counseling, psychotherapy, biofeedback, stress reduction, colon therapy, a weight reduction program, anti-smoking therapy, pain management, a wellness program, and homeopathy.

Robbie Davis-Floyd, an anthropologist, and Gloria St. John, who has worked as a health administrator and consultant, conducted intensive interviews with 34 holistic physicians. None of their subjects were AMA members, and most were not members of state, county, or local medical societies (Davis-Floyd and St. John 1998:208). Davis-Floyd and St. John delineated the following factors that prompted physicians to make a paradigm shift from biomedicine, or "technocratic medicine," to holistic medicine: (1) an experience with the limits of biomedicine; (2) an encounter with a patient who informed them about the merits of holistic medicine; (3) a personal illness that biomedicine could not adequately treat; and (4) a social and spiritual experience that altered their relationship with friends, family, and society (Davis-Floyd and St. John 1998:150–69). While the holistic physicians in the study encountered animosity from some of their biomedical colleagues, they also received the admiration of other colleagues for their decision to embrace holistic medicine.

Despite the growing interest of biomedical and osteopathic physicians in holistic health, it is important to remember, as Alster so aptly observes, "that physicians were latecomers, arriving to find other groups already well established and claiming to offer different and even superior services than those available from physicians or physician-controlled agencies" (1989:161). Within the corridors of biomedicine itself, nurses, occupational therapists, and physical therapists expressed an interest in holistic health well before physicians did. While undoubtedly some biomedical physicians are genuinely sympathetic to holistic and alternative approaches, patients and other health professionals appear to have created the climate that demanded that an increasing number of biomedical physicians give serious consideration to the holistic health movement.

In keeping with the general tendency of nurses to be "person-oriented" rather than "disease-oriented," as biomedical physicians tend to be, it should not be surprising that the former have responded much more favorably to alternative medical systems than have the latter. The American Holistic Nurses' Association was formed in 1980 and is presently headquartered in Flagstaff, Arizona. Keegan maintains that "this organization has encouraged nurses to adopt the role of healer and seek to tighten the loosened threads of body, mind, and spirit" (1988:68). Holistic nurses have expressed an interest in environmental protection, relaxation techniques, imagery, music therapy, and touch therapy.

Although some M.D.s and D.O.s subscribe to the philosophical underpinnings of various heterodox medical systems, others adopt their techniques without wholeheartedly subscribing to their ideologies. Kotarba (1983) argues that the incorporation of holistic principles into NASA's comprehensive health program was designed to optimize work performance but that the agency did not adopt an organizational commitment to the overall ideology of the holistic health movement. Despite the claim on the part of holistic health proponents that they wish to contribute to a process of demedicalization by shifting responsibility for health care from the physician to the patient, the growing emphasis on the holistic model within biomedicine may actually be contributing to further medicalization in American society. The holistic health movement runs the risk of becoming a subtle moral crusade which equates specific lifestyles with moral failures and in essence depoliticizes the social origins of disease by blaming the victim (Crawford 1977; Lowenberg 1989). As Lowenberg and Davis (1994:592) observe, "holistic health practice ultimately extends the control of medical definitions and even gatekeeping to incorporate far wider arenas of lifestyle, spirituality, work, and family."

GROWING CORPORATE AND GOVERNMENTAL INTEREST
IN ALTERNATIVE MEDICINE

Much of the recent corporate and governmental interest in alternative medicine is due to efforts at cost containment. As a result of a congressional mandate, the National Institutes of Health (NIH) established an Office of Alternative Medicine (OAM) in 1992. The office reportedly was created "under pressure from a Congress alarmed by the soaring costs of high-tech healing and the frustrating fact that so many ailments—AIDS, cancer, arthritis, back pain—have yet to yield to standard medicine" (Toufexis 1993:43). OAM has been designated to explore the efficacy of selected heterodox therapies. The OAM's annual budget has steadily increased, from $2 million in fiscal year (FY) 1992 to $50 million in FY 1999. These figures are minuscule, however, in comparison to the annual budget of the National Institutes of Health, which was set at $13.648 billion for FY 1998.

While the OAM has provided alternative medicine with high visibility and a certain legitimacy, it appears to be inadvertently contributing to the biomedical co-optation of the holistic health movement. According to Nienstedt,

> What could have been a ground-breaking opportunity for alternative medicine practitioners to gain official respectability for their professions while maintaining their ideological integrity have [sic] not materialized. Instead, there appears to be an effort by the OAM to entice biomedicine into leadership in the agency by invitations to participate in key roles and bestow their approval to alternatives. (Nienstedt 1998:39)

The OAM Advisory Council was headed by Wayne Jonas, a biomedical physician on a three-year leave from the Walter Reed Army Institute of Research. The council consists of 18 members—research scientists, health practitioners, and other interested parties, most of whom have a biomedical orientation. Of the 13 Specialty Research Centers that have received funding, 11 are located at large biomedical institutions: the medical schools at the University of Virginia; Columbia University; the University of Maryland; the University of California, Davis; Stanford University; the University of Medicine and Dentistry, New Jersey; the University of Texas, Houston; the University of Arizona; the University of Michigan; the University of Minnesota; and Harvard University. Bastyr University—a naturopathic institution—and the Palmer Center for Chiropractic Research in Davenport, Iowa, are the only alternative institutions funded by OAM. Each research site investigates the efficacy and safety of alternative therapies for various diseases or health problems, such as asthma, AIDS, cancer, stroke, cardiovascular complications, and drug addiction.

Most of the interest on the part of corporations and government agencies has been directed toward therapies that fall under the general rubric of the holistic health/New Age movement. Adherents of this movement have been better positioned to receive a hearing from strategic elites than have working-class people of color who often rely upon folk medical systems. Whereas the holistic health movement has evolved into a source of alternative therapies for upper-class and middle-class people, folk medical systems continue to cater to working-class European Americans, African Americans, Haitian Americans, Hispanic Americans, Asian Americans, and Native Americans.

THE PERSISTENCE OF FOLK MEDICAL SYSTEMS IN THE CONTEXT OF BIOMEDICAL DOMINATION

Although most working-class people, including those of color, rely primarily on biomedicine for health care, it appears that folk medical beliefs and practices persist, and in some instances even are being revitalized, not only among Native Americans but among other ethnic minorities in the United States. Many African Americans, particularly those belonging to the working class, continue to rely on folk medical remedies and on healers who treat not only physical ailments but also emotional problems stemming from racism and poverty. Bailey (1991) found among a sample of African Americans in Detroit that 24 percent of the women and about 10 percent of the men reported using folk or "personal" care treatments for hypertension. Despite the persistence of folk medical systems, scholars have, for the most part, only an impressionistic sense of how widespread they are in American society. Snow (1993:265–69) ascribes the persistence of African American folk medicine to three factors: the poor treatment of blacks in biomedical settings; economic deprivation, which often makes quality biomedical care unavailable; and the patients' search for a greater sense of control over their lives. Watson argues that,

> The widespread development and persistence of traditional medicine among Afro-Americans and their corresponding underutilization of modern medical practitioners are largely traceable to economic poverty, ignorance, and poor health. In particular, the history of racism and segregation in public accommodations in the United States has helped to produce low rates of Afro-American uses of modern health care facilities. (Watson 1984:53) ["Ignorance" would be better phrased as lack of access to information.]

Some time ago, Trotter and Chavira (1981) asserted that curanderismo was undergoing a period of efflorescence in the Lower Rio Grande Valley. Rivera (1988) reported that 32 percent of Mexican Americans in urban barrios in Colorado sought health care from curandero/as. In a survey of 2,103 people born in Mexico but living or working in San Diego, Chavez (1984:34) found that only 27 (1.3 percent) reported that they had actually used a curandera or curandero, but 429 (23.3 percent) expressed willingness to do so. Many Puerto Ricans rely at one time or other during their lives on the services of espiritistas (Garrison 1977a; Singer and Borrero 1984; Harwood 1987).

There has been an overall decline of traditional healers among Native Americans, despite the persistence of Native American medical beliefs. With the encroachment of non-native settlers, shamanism underwent a rapid decline among the Washo Indians of the Intermountain West. Siskin (1983:171–72) reported that only ten Washo shamans remained in 1939, and in 1956 there was only one, Henry Rupert, who died in 1973. Rupert, who spent much of his life in European American society as a printer, hypnotist, farmer, and entrepreneur, incorporated Hindu and Hawaiian personages into his pantheon of spirit guides and was the first Washo healer to eschew a belief in sorcery. John Frank, a Washo healer who was in his nineties in the early 1980s, was never in Siskin's (1983:201) opinion a "full-fledged shaman"; he was an elderly man when he began to doctor in 1974 after having watched Rupert cure over the years.

Based upon her research among the Eastern Band of Cherokee in the Smoky Mountains region of western North Carolina, Kupferer (1972:296) reported that traditional Indians continued to rely upon "Indian doctors" but generally combined Cherokee medicine with biomedicine. Some elderly Cherokees attempted to restrict themselves to native healers because "they believe that the hospital is a place where people die" (Kupferer 1972:296). Kunitz and Levy reported a general decline of Navajo singers on the Kaibito Plateau:

> In 1905 there were twenty ceremonialists on the Kaibito Plateau and there was a ratio of one ceremonialist to thirty patients. By the 1950s the number had increased to forty-eight but, with the rapidly increasing population, there were fifty patients to each ceremonialist. By 1980 there were only twenty-four ceremonialists serving a population of 4,244, a ratio of 1:176. . . . Not only has the number of ceremonialists declined but so has the number of different ceremonies. (1997: 116–17)

In response to the decline of singers on the Navajo reservation, the Navajo Nation Medicinemen's Association established a school that trains singers. Anthropologist Donald Bahr estimated the presence of some 150 shamans among the Pima Indians of southern Arizona during the early 1970s (Bahr et al. 1974).

People of color are integrating their traditional medical systems with other alternative therapies, such as chiropractic, naturopathy, acupuncture, massage, yoga, tai chi, and meditation. According to Semmes, the adoption of such "naturalistic health practices" by African Americans constitutes an effort to rejuvenate earlier traditional African medicine:

> They perpetuate the view that health is a function of interpersonal, spiritual, and ecological equilibrium. Naturalistic health practices tend to revitalize and pre- serve [the] African and African-American tradition that health is fundamentally religious and connected to how God wants you to live. (1996:103)

In response to numerous critiques asserting that biomedicine tends to be insensitive to cultural diversity, many medical schools and some hospitals have made efforts to acquaint their health workers with the health beliefs and practices of patients belonging to various ethnic minorities. Some biomedi- cal centers, particularly those associated with medical schools, and Indian Health Service hospitals have entered into a "therapeutic alliance" with folk or indigenous healers. While such arrangements have served to make bio- medical practitioners more sensitive to the cultural background of minority patients, they have not seriously challenged biomedical hegemony. Indeed, Philip Singer views the "therapeutic alliance" as a manifestation of a "new colonialism," contending that under this arrangement, individual healing me- diates between the individual and the hegemonic institutions with which he or she has to struggle (Singer 1977:17–20). He maintains that medical anthro- pologists who collaborate with biomedical practitioners, particularly psychia- trists, within the context of the "therapeutic alliance" contribute to the status quo by reinforcing a therapeutic system that provides symptom relief rather than eradication of illness. Although Trotter and Chavira do not object to the notion of a "therapeutic alliance" per se, they express serious concern about efforts to integrate Mexican American curanderos into biomedical health set- tings:

> In their own communities, *curanderos* are the equivalent of the highest-ranking therapists. . . . Would they be accepted into the medical system on an equal status with the physician and clinical psychologist? Unlikely! They probably would be brought in as orderlies, assistants, or in some other low-status position. (1981:170)

An emancipatory "therapeutic alliance" would require an egalitarian relation- ship between representatives of different medical systems, one that would transcend the hierarchical structure of the American dominative medical sys- tem. Indeed, Marc Micozzi, the executive director of the College of Physi- cians in Philadelphia and the founding editor of the *Journal of Alternative and Complementary Medicine,* calls for "tolerance and medical pluralism" as well as a shift in power relationships between physician and patient (Redwood 1995:1).

TOWARD AN AUTHENTICALLY HOLISTIC AND
PLURALISTIC MEDICAL SYSTEM

Some social scientists have argued that the holistic health movement contains the potential of serving as a medical "countersystem." Lyng, for example, asserts that

> A basic tenet of holistic health thinking is that no one body of medical knowledge can take into account all aspects of health reality, and, therefore, all medical perspectives are aspects of health reality, and, therefore, all medical perspectives are inherently partial. Consequently, the only way to deal with all of the different facets of health reality is to adopt a multitherapeutic approach, which, in turn, demands a multiperspectival system. (1990:94)

While the type of holistic and pluralistic medical countersystem that Lyng proposes is an ideal worth striving for, it is important to reiterate that the holistic health movement by and large has adopted a limited holism that stresses mind-body connections but fails to make adequate mind-body-society connections. Indeed, its proponents all too often use the notion of holistic health as a rhetorical device that serves their own ends, including professional and pecuniary ones, rather than as a substantive one that could provide a critique of the existing American political economy and its associated dominative medical system (Hufford and Chilton 1996:63). The holistic health movement caters to a largely white, middle-class clientele and has failed to reach out to working-class and racial/ethnic minorities in American society.

The creation of an authentically holistic and pluralistic medical system ultimately will have to be coupled with the demand for a universal health care system, one that incorporates alternative therapies and that treats health care as a right rather than a privilege. As Flacks (1993:465) argues, "the demand for a universal health-care program . . . has the potential to politically unite very diverse movement constituencies and to link these with middle-class voters." Both of these efforts will need to be part and parcel of a yet larger effort that seeks to transcend capitalism not only at the national level but at the global level and to replace it with a global system of democratic eco-socialism (Baer, Singer, and Susser 1997:232–34). Democratic eco-socialism is based on the following principles: (1) public ownership of a predominant part of the economy, (2) egalitarianism, (3) workers' democracy, (4) a combination of centralized and decentralized social structures, and (5) a recognition that we live on an ecologically fragile planet with limited resources that must be sustained and renewed for future generations. It constitutes a vision entailing a prolonged process of struggle that will meet with resistance from the corporate class and its political allies for some time to come. For the immediate future, progressives need to focus on concrete issues concerning various human social needs including health and the eradication of disease, both of which may be met in part by biomedicine and an array of alternative healing systems.

Bibliography
Index

Bibliography

Abrams, Maxine. 1994. Alternate medicine: Quackery or miracle? *Good Housekeeping*, March, 99–119.

Alabama State Chiropractic Association. 1993. *The cost effectiveness of chiropractic*. Montgomery: Alabama State Chiropractic Association.

Albanese, Catherine L. 1986. Physic and metaphysic in nineteenth-century America: Medical sectarians and religious healing. *Church History* 55:489–502.

Albanese, Catherine L. 1990. *Nature religion in America: From the Algonkian Indians to the New Age*. Chicago: University of Chicago Press.

Albrecht, Gary L., and Judith A. Levy. 1982. The professionalization of osteopathy: Adaptation in the medical marketplace. In *Research in the sociology of health care*, vol. 2: *Changing structure of health service occupations*, ed. Julius A. Roth, 161–206. Greenwich, Conn.: JAI Press.

Alexander, Kay. 1992. Roots of the New Age. In *Perspectives on the New Age*, ed. James R. Lewis and J. Gordon Melton, 30–47. Albany: State University of New York Press.

Alford, Robert. 1972. The political economy of health care: Dynamics without change. *Politics and Society* 2:127–64.

Alster, Kristine Beyerman. 1989. *The holistic health movement*. Tuscaloosa: University of Alabama Press.

American Chiropractic Association. 1983. Working together for the benefit of chiropractic. *ACA Journal of Chiropractic* 20(10):18–26.

American Medical Association. 1955. Report of the Committee for the Study of Relations between Osteopathy and Medicine. *Journal of the American Medical Association* 158:736–41.

American Medical Association. 1959. Digest of official actions, 1846–1958. Chicago.

American Osteopathic Association. 1902. Report of the Committee for Education. *Journal of the American Osteopathic Association* 2:10–19.

Anderson, Robert Mapes. 1979. *Vision of the disinherited: The making of American Pentecostalism*. New York: Oxford University Press.

Anderson, Robert T. 1981. Medicine, chiropractic, and caste. *Anthropological Quarterly* 54:157–65.

Anderson, Robert T. 1987. The treatment of musculoskeletal disorders by a Mexican bonesetter (*sobador*). *Social Science and Medicine* 24:43–46.

193

Anderson, Robert T. 1991. An American clinic for traditional Chinese medicine: Comparisons to family medicine and chiropractic. *Journal of Manipulative and Physiological Therapeutics* 14(8):462–66.

Atkinson, Jane Monnig. 1992. Shamanisms today. *Annual Review of Anthropology* 21: 307–30.

Babbie, Earl. 1990. Channels to elsewhere. In *In gods we trust: New patterns of religious pluralism in America.* 2d ed. Ed. Thomas Robbins and Dick Anthony, 255–68. New Brunswick, N.J.: Transaction Publishers.

Baer, Hans A. 1981a. Prophets and advisors in black Spiritual churches: Therapy, palliative, or opiate. *Culture, Medicine and Psychiatry* 5:145–70.

Baer, Hans A. 1981b. The organization rejuvenation of osteopathy: A reflection of the decline of professional dominance in medicine. *Social Science and Medicine* 15A:701–11.

Baer, Hans A. 1982. Toward a typology of black folk healers. *Phylon* 43:327–43.

Baer, Hans A. 1984a. *The black Spiritual movement: A religious response to racism.* Knoxville: University of Tennessee Press.

Baer, Hans A. 1984b. The drive for professionalization in British osteopathy. *Social Science and Medicine* 19:717–25.

Baer, Hans A. 1984c. A comparative view of a heterodox system: Chiropractic in America and Britain. *Medical Anthropology* 8:151–68.

Baer, Hans A. 1989. The American dominative medical system as a reflection of social relations in the larger society. *Social Science and Medicine* 28:1103–12.

Baer, Hans A. 1996. Practice-building seminars in chiropractic: A petit bourgeois response to biomedical domination. *Medical Anthropology Quarterly* 10:29–44.

Baer, Hans A., and Merrill Singer. 1992. *African-American religion in the twentieth century: Varieties of protest and accommodation.* Knoxville: University of Tennessee Press.

Baer, Hans A., Merrill Singer, and Ida Susser. 1997. *Medical anthropology and the world system: A critical perspective.* Westport, Conn.: Bergin and Garvey.

Baer, Leonard D., and Charles M. Good, Jr. 1998. The power of the state. In *Alternative therapies: Expanding options in health care,* ed. Rena J. Gordon, Barbara Cable, and Wilbert M. Gesler, 45–66. New York: Springer Publishing Company.

Bahr, Donald M., Juan Gregorio, David I. Lopez, and Albert Alvarez. 1974. *Piman shamanism and staying sickness.* Tucson: University of Arizona Press.

Bailey, Eric J. 1991. Hypertension: An analysis of Detroit African American health care treatment patterns. *Human Organization* 50:287–96.

Barash, Douglas S. 1992. The mainstreaming of alternative medicine. *New York Times Magazine,* October 4, 6–9 and 36–38.

Barnes, Linda L. 1998. The psychologizing of Chinese healing practices in the United States. *Culture, Medicine and Psychiatry* 22:413–43.

Barnes, Margaret W. 1971. History of the Academy of Applied Osteopathy. In *1971 Yearbook of selected osteopathic papers.* American Academy of Osteopathy, 57–73.

Barrett, Stephen. 1976. The unhealthy alliance. In *The health robbers: How to protect your money and your life,* ed. Stephen Barrett and Gilda Knight, 189–201. Philadelphia: George F. Stickley.

194

Bass, Ruth. 1981. Mojo. In *Mother wit from the laughing barrel: Readings in the interpretation of Afro-American folklore,* ed. Alan Dundes, 380–87. New York: Garland.

Bednarowski, Mary Farrell. 1995. The Church of Scientology: Lightning rod for cultural boundary conflicts. In *America's alternative religions,* ed. Timothy Miller, 385–92. Albany: State University of New York.

Bergemann, Brian W., and Anthony J. Cichoke. 1980. Cost-effectiveness of medical vs. chiropractic treatment of low-back injuries. *Journal of Manipulative and Physiological Therapeutics* 3(3):143–47.

Bergman, Jerry. 1995. The Adventist and Jehovah's Witness branch of Protestantism. In *America's alternative religions,* ed. Timothy Miller, 33–46. Albany: State University of New York.

Berliner, Howard S. 1975. A larger perspective on the Flexner Report. *International Journal of Health Services* 5:573–92.

Berliner, Howard S. 1982. Medical modes of production. In *The problem of medical knowledge: Examining the social construction of medicine,* ed. Andrew Treacher and Peter Wright, 162–73. Edinburgh: Edinburgh University Press.

Berliner, Howard S. 1985. *A system of scientific medicine: Philanthropic foundations in the Flexner era.* New York: Tavistock Publications.

Berliner, Howard, and J. Warren Salmon. 1979. The holistic health movement and scientific medicine: The naked and the dead. *Socialist Review* 43:31–52.

Berliner, Howard, and J. Warren Salmon. 1980. The holistic alternative to scientific medicine: History and analysis. *International Journal of Health Services* 10:133–47.

Berman, Alex. 1956. Neo-Thomsonianism in the United States. *Journal of the History of Medicine and Allied Sciences* 11:133–44.

Berman, Alex. 1978. The heroic approach in nineteenth-century therapeutics. In *Sickness and health in America: Readings in the history of medicine and public health.* 1st ed. Ed. Judith Walzer Leavitt and Ronald L. Numbers, 77–86. Madison: University of Wisconsin Press.

Blackstone, Erwin A. 1977. The AMA and the osteopaths: A study of the power of organized medicine. *Antitrust Bulletin* 22:405–40.

Bloom, Harold. 1992. *The American religion: The emergence of the post-Christian nation.* New York: Simon and Schuster.

Bloomfield, Robert J. 1983. Naturopathy. In *Traditional medicine and health care coverage: A reader for health administrators and practitioners,* ed. Robert H. Bannerman, John Burton, and Ch'en Wen-Chieh, 116–23. Geneva: World Health Organization.

Bocock, Robert. 1986. *Hegemony.* London: Tavistock.

Booth, E. R. 1924. *History of osteopathy and twentieth-century medical practice.* Cincinnati: Caxton.

Bord, Richard J., and Joseph E. Faulkner. 1983. *The Catholic Charismatics: The anatomy of a modern religious movement.* University Park: Pennsylvania State University.

Borre, Kristen S., and James L. Wilson. 1998. Paradigms and politics: Redux of homeopathy in American medicine. *Alternative therapies: Expanding options in health care,* ed. Rena J. Gordon, Barbara Cable Nienstedt, and Wilbert M. Gesler, 67–84. New York: Springer Publishing Company.

Bourgeault, Ivy Lynn, and Mary Fynes. 1997. Integrating lay and nurse-midwifery into the U.S. and Canadian health care systems. *Social Science and Medicine* 44: 1051–63.

Brandon, George. 1990. Sacrificial practices in santeria, an African-Cuban religion in the United States. In *Africanisms in American culture*, ed. Joseph E. Holloway, 119–47. Bloomington: Indiana University Press.

Brandon, George. 1991. The uses of plants in healing in Afro-Cuban religion, santeria. *Journal of Black Studies* 22:55–76.

Brandon, George. 1993. *Santeria from Africa to the New World: The dead sell memories.* Bloomington: Indiana University Press.

Bratman, Steven. 1997. *The alternative medicine sourcebook: A realistic evaluation of alternative healing systems.* Chicago: Contemporary Books.

Braude, Ann. 1989. *Radical spirits: Spiritualism and women's rights in nineteenth-century America.* Boston: Beacon Press.

Bromley, David G., and Mitchell L. Bracey, Jr. 1998. The Church of Scientology: A quasi-religion. In *Sects, cults, and spiritual communities: A sociological analysis*, ed. William W. Zellner and Marc Petrowsky, 141–56. Boulder, Colo.: Westview Press.

Brown, David H. 1990. Conjure/doctors: An exploration of a black discourse in America, antebellum to 1940. *Folklore Forum* 23(1/2):3–46.

Brown, E. Richard. 1979. *Rockefeller medicine men: Medicine and capitalism in America.* Berkeley: University of California Press.

Brown, Karen McCarthy. 1991. *Mama Lola: A vodou priestess in Brooklyn.* Berkeley: University of California Press.

Brown, Michael F. 1997. *The channeling zone: American spirituality in an anxious age.* Cambridge, Mass.: Harvard University Press.

Brown, P. R. 1987. Social context and medical theory in the demarcation of nineteenth-century boundaries. In *Medical fringe and medical orthodoxy, 1750–1850*, ed. W. F. Bynum and Roy Porter, 216–33. London: Croom Helm.

Bucko, Raymond A. 1998. *The Lakota ritual of the sweat lodge: History and contemporary practice.* Lincoln: University of Nebraska Press.

Burrow, James Gordon. 1963. *AMA: Voice of American medicine.* Baltimore: Johns Hopkins Press.

Butler, Kurt. 1992. *A consumer's guide to "alternative medicine."* Buffalo: Prometheus Books.

Campbell, Gary H. 1979. The vanishing osteopathic physician. *Osteopathic Medicine* 4(9):17–20.

Caplan, Ronald L. 1991. Health-care reform and chiropractic in the 1990s. *Journal of Manipulative and Physiological Therapeutics* 14:341–54.

Capps, Lisa L. 1994. Change and continuity in the medical culture of the Hmong in Kansas City. *Medical Anthropology Quarterly* 8:161–77.

Cargill, Marie. 1994. *Acupuncture: A viable medical alternative.* Westport, Conn.: Praeger.

Carter, James P. 1993. *Racketeering in medicine: The suppression of alternatives.* Norfolk, Va.: Hampton Roads Publishing.

Cavender, Anthony P., and Scott H. Beck. 1995. Generational change, folk medicine, and medical self-care in a rural Appalachian community. *Human Organization* 54: 129–42.

Cayleff, Susan E. 1988. Gender, ideology, and the water-cure movement. In *Other healers: Unorthodox medicine in America,* ed. Norman Gevitz, 82–98. Baltimore: Johns Hopkins University Press.

Chavez, Leo R. 1984. Doctors, curanderos, and brujas: Health care delivery and Mexican immigrants in San Diego. *Medical Anthropology Quarterly* 15(2):31–37.

Chopra, Deepak. 1990. *Perfect health: The complete mind-body guide.* Harmony: Crown.

Chow, Effie Poy Yew. 1984. Traditional Chinese medicine: A holistic system. In *Alternative medicines: Popular and policy perspectives,* ed. J. Warren Salmon, 114–37. New York: Tavistock.

Christian Science Publishing Society. 1990. *Christian Science: A sourcebook of contemporary materials.* Boston: The Christian Science Publishing Society.

Churchill, W., and W. LaDuke. 1985. Radioactive colonization and Native Americans. *Socialist Review* 81:95–199.

Citizens Committee on Education for Health Care. 1967. Osteopathy in the United States and Michigan: A staff report from the Citizens on Education for Health Care for presentation to the state board for health care.

Clark, Margaret. 1970. *Health in the Mexican-American culture: A community study.* 2d ed. Berkeley: University of California Press.

Clark, Mary Ann. 1998. Santeria. In *Sects, cults, and spiritual communities: A sociological analysis,* ed. William W. Zellner and Marc Petrowsky, 117–30. Boulder, Colo.: Westview Press.

Clarkson, Frederick. 1997. *Eternal hostility: The struggle between theocracy and democracy.* Monroe, Maine: Common Courage Press.

Cobb, Ann Kuckelman. 1981. Incorporation and change: The case of the midwife in the United States. *Medical Anthropology* 5:73–88.

Cobbins, Otho B. 1966. *History of Church of Christ (Holiness) U.S.A., 1895–1965.* New York: Vantage Press.

Coburn, David, and C. Lesley Biggs. 1986. Limits to medical dominance: The case of chiropractic. *Social Science and Medicine* 22:1035–46.

Cockerham, William C. 1995. *Medical sociology.* Englewood Cliffs, N.J.: Prentice-Hall.

Cody, George. 1985. History of naturopathic medicine. In *A textbook of natural medicine,* ed. J. E. Pizzorno and M. T. Murray, 1–24. Seattle: John Bastyr College Publications.

Cohen, Marcine. 1983. Medical social movements in the United States (1820–1982): The case of osteopathy. Ph.D. dissertation, University of California, San Digeo.

Cohen, Wilbur J. 1968. Independent practitioners under Medicare: A report to the Congress. Washington, D.C.: U.S. Department of Health, Education, and Welfare.

Collinge, William. 1996. *The American Holistic Health Association complete guide to alternative medicine.* New York: Time Warner Books.

Cooley, Gilbert E. 1977. Root doctors and psychics in the region. *Indiana Folklore* 10: 191–200.

Cooper, Gregory S. 1985. The attitude of organized medicine toward chiropractic: A sociohistorical perspective. *Chiropractic History* 5:19–25.

197

Cooter, Roger. 1988. Alternative medicine, alternative cosmology. In *Studies in the history of alternative medicine,* ed. Roger Cooter, 63–78. New York: St. Martin's Press.

Coulehan, John L. 1985a. Chiropractic and the clinical art. *Social Science and Medicine* 21:383–90.

Coulehan, John L. 1985b. Adjustment, the hands and healing. *Culture, Medicine and Psychiatry* 9:353–82.

Coulter, Harris L. 1973. *Divided legacy: A history of the schism in medical thought,* vol. 3: *Science and ethics in American medicine, 1800–1914.* Washington, D.C.: Wehawken.

Coulter, Harris L. 1984. Homeopathy. In *Alternative medicines: Popular and policy perspectives,* ed. J. Warren Salmon, 57–79. New York: Tavistock.

Coulter, Ian D., Ron D. Hays, and Clark D. Danielson. 1996. The role of the chiropractor in the changing health care system: From marginal to mainstream. In *Research in the sociology of health care,* vol. 13A: *Health care delivery system changes,* ed. Jennie J. Kronenfeld, 95–117. Greenwich, Conn.: JAI Press.

Cowie, James B., and Julian Roebuck. 1975. *An ethnography of a chiropractic clinic.* New York: Free Press.

Crawford, Nelson Antrim. 1962. "Consult with D.O.s? We've done it for years." *Medical Economics,* March 12, 236–50.

Crawford, Robert. 1977. You are dangerous to your health: The ideology and politics of victim blaming. *International Journal of Health Services* 7:663–80.

Croon, Edward M., Jr. 1992. Herbal medicine among the Lumbee Indians. In *Herbal and magical medicine: Traditional healing today,* ed. James Kirkland et al., 137–69. Durham, N.C.: Duke University Press.

Csordas, Thomas J. 1983. The rhetoric of transformation in ritual healing. *Culture, Medicine and Psychiatry* 7:333–75.

Csordas, Thomas J. 1994. *The sacred self: A cultural phenomenology of charismatic healing.* Berkeley: University of California Press.

Cunningham, Raymond J. 1974. From holiness to healing: The faith cure in America, 1872–1892. *Church History* 43:499–513.

Curry, Mary Cuthrell. 1997. *Making the gods in New York: The Yoruba religion in the African American community.* New York: Garland Publishing.

Danforth, Loring M. 1989. *Firewalking and religious healing: The Anastenaria of Greece and the American firewalking movement.* Princeton, N.J.: Princeton University Press.

D'Andrade, Hugh. 1974. *Charles Fillmore: Herald of the New Age.* New York: Harper and Row.

D'Antonio, Michael. 1992. *Heaven on earth.* New York: Crown Publishers.

Davis-Floyd, Robbie, and Gloria St. John. 1998. *From doctor to healer: The transformative journey.* New Brunswick, N.J.: Rutgers University Press.

de Chant, Dell. 1993. Myrtle Fillmore and her daughters: An observation and analysis of the role of women in Unity. In *Women's leadership in marginal religions: Explorations outside the mainstream,* ed. Catherine Wessinger, 102–24. Urbana: University of Illinois Press.

DeHood, N. B. 1937. The diffusion of a system of belief. Ph.D. dissertation, Harvard University.

Delp, Robert W. 1987. Andrew Jackson Davis and Spiritualism. In *Pseudo-science and society in nineteenth-century America,* ed. Arthur Wrobel, 100–121. Lexington: University Press of Kentucky.

Denbow, C. 1977. Osteopathy: Packing more professional punch. *Medical Opinions,* May 19, 19–24.

Densmore, Frances. 1974. *How Indians use wild plants for food, medicine and crafts.* New York: Dover Publications.

Derber, Charles. 1983. Sponsorship and the control of physicians. *Theory and Society* 12:561–601.

DeVries, Raymond G. 1982. Midwifery and the problem of licensure. In *Research in the sociology of health care,* vol. 2: *Changing structure of health service occupations,* ed. Julius A. Roth, 77–120. Greenwich, Conn.: JAI Press.

DeVries, Raymond G. 1993. A cross-national view of the status of midwives. In *Gender, work, and medicine: Women and the medical division of labor,* ed. Elianne Riska and Katarina Weger, 131–46. London: Sage Publications.

The D.O.: growing pains. 1980. *Medical World News* 21(2):42–51.

Domhoff, G. William. 1967. *Who rules America?* Englewood Cliffs, N.J.: Prentice-Hall.

Domhoff, G. William. 1990. *The power elite and the state: How policy is made in America.* New York: Aldine de Gruyter.

Dougherty, Molly C. 1982. Southern midwifery and organized health care: Systems in conflict. *Medical Anthropology* 6:114–26.

Droogers, Andre. 1994. The normalization of religious experience: Healing, prophecy, dreams, and visions. In *Charismatic Christianity as a global culture,* ed. Karla Poewe, 33–49. Columbia: University of South Carolina Press.

Duffy, D. J. 1978. *A study of Wisconsin industrial back injury and neck injuries, 1976–77.* Des Moines: Iowa Industrial Commission.

Duffy, John. 1976. *The healers: A history of American medicine.* Urbana: University of Illinois Press.

Eckberg, Douglas Lee. 1987. The dilemma of osteopathic physicians and the rationalization of medical practice. *Social Science and Medicine* 25:1111–20.

Ehrenreich, Barbara, and John Ehrenreich. 1970. *The American health empire: Power, profits, and politics.* New York: Random House.

Ehrenreich, Barbara, and John Ehrenreich. 1978. Medicine and social control. In *The cultural crisis of modern medicine,* ed. John Ehrenreich, Pp. 39–79. New York: Monthly Review Press.

Eisenberg, David M., et al. 1993. Unconventional medicine in the United States. *New England Journal of Medicine* 328(4):246–52.

Eisenberg, David M., et al. 1998. Trends in alternative medicine use in the United States, 1990–1997: Results of a follow-up national study. *Journal of the American Medical Association* 280(18):1569–75.

Elling, Ray. 1981. The political economy, cultural hegemony, and mixes of traditional and modern medicine. *Social Science and Medicine* 15A:89–99.

Ellwood, Robert S. 1973. *Religious and spiritual groups in modern America*. Englewood Cliffs, N.J.: Prentice-Hall.

English-Lueck, J. A. 1990. *Health in the new age: A study in California holistic practices*. Albuquerque: University of New Mexico Press.

Evans, E. Raymond, Clive Kileff, and Karen Shelley. 1982. *Herbal medicine: A living force in the Appalachians*. Durham, N.C.: Medical History Program and the Trent Collection.

Femia, Joseph V. 1981. *Gramsci's political thought: Hegemony, consciousness, and the revolutionary process*. Oxford: Clarendon Press.

Finken, D. 1986. Naturopathy: America's homegrown alternative healing art. *Medical Self-Care* (November/December):39–43.

Finkler, Kaja. 1985. *Spiritualist healers in Mexico: Successes and failures of alternative therapeutics*. South Hadley, Mass.: Bergin and Garvey Publishers.

Fishbein, Morris. 1932. *Medical follies*. New York: Boni and Liveright.

Fishman, Robert Gart. 1979. Spiritualism in western New York: A study in ritual healing. *Medical Anthropology* 3:1–23.

Flacks, Richard. 1993. The party's over—so what is to be done? *Social Research* 60: 445–70.

Foundation for the Advancement of Chiropractic Tenets and Science. 1980. *Chiropractic health care*, vol. 1: *A national health study of cost of education, service utilization, number of practicing doctors of chiropractic and other key policy issues*. Washington, D.C.: FACTS.

Foster, George M., and Barbara Gallatin Anderson. 1978. *Medical anthropology*. New York: John Wiley and Sons.

Fox, Margery. 1989. The socioreligious role of the Christian Science practitioner. In *Women as healers: Cross-cultural perspectives*, ed. Carol Shepherd McClain, 98–115. New Brunswick, N.J.: Rutgers University Press.

Frankenberg, Ronald. 1981. Allopathic medicine, profession, and capitalist ideology in India. *Social Science and Medicine* 15A:115–25.

Freidson, Eliot. 1970. *Profession of medicine: A study of the sociology of applied knowledge*. New York: Harper and Row.

Fugh-Berman, Adriane. 1993. "Natural" medicine. *The Nation*, September 6/13, 240–45.

Fuller, Robert C. 1989. *Alternative medicine and American religious life*. New York: Oxford University Press.

Gardner, Martin. 1957. *Fads and fallacies in the name of science*. New York: Dover.

Garrison, Vivian. 1977a. Doctor, *espiritista*, or psychiatrist? Health-seeking behavior in a Puerto Rican neighborhood of New York City. *Medical Anthropology* 2:65–191.

Garrison, Vivian. 1977b. The "Puerto Rican syndrome" in psychiatry and *espiritismo*. In *Case studies in spirit possession*, ed. Vincent Crapanzano and Vivian Garrison, 383–449. New York: John Wiley and Sons.

Genovese, Eugene D. 1974. *Roll, Jordan, roll: The world the slaves made*. New York: Vintage Books.

Gesler, Wilbert M., and Rena J. Gordon. 1998. Alternative therapies: Why now? In *Alternative therapies: Expanding options in health care*, ed. Rena J. Gordon, Barbara Cable Nienstedt, and Wilbert M. Gesler, 3–24. New York: Springer Publishing Company.

Gevitz, Norman. 1982. *The D.O.s: Osteopathic medicine in America.* Baltimore: Johns Hopkins University Press.

Gevitz, Norman. 1988a. "A coarse sieve": Basic science boards and medical licensure in the United States. *Journal of the History of Medicine and Allied Sciences* 43:36–63.

Gevitz, Norman. 1988b. Osteopathic medicine: From deviance to difference. In *Other healers: Unorthodox medicine in America,* ed. Norman Gevitz, 124–56. Baltimore: Johns Hopkins University Press.

Gevitz, Norman. 1992. The fate of sectarian medical education. In *Beyond Flexner: Medical education in the twentieth century,* ed. Barbara Barzansky and Norman Gevitz, 83–97. New York: Greenwood Press.

Gibbons, Russell W. 1977. Chiropractic history: Turbulence and triumph—the survival of a profession. In *Who's who in chiropractic, international, 1976–78,* ed. Fern L. Dzaman, 138–48. Littleton, Colo.: Who's Who in Chiropractic, International Publishing.

Gibbons, Russell W. 1980. The evolution of chiropractic: Medical and social protest in America. In *Modern developments in the principles and practice of chiropractic,* ed. Scott Haldeman, 3–24. New York: Appleton and Lange.

Gibbons, Russell W. 1981. Physician-chiropractors: Medical presence in the evolution of chiropractic. *Bulletin of the History of Medicine* 55:233–45.

Gibbons, Russell W. 1982. Forgotten parameters of general practice: The chiropractic obstetrician. *Chiropractic History* 2(1):27–34.

Gill, Gillian. 1998. *Mary Baker Eddy.* Reading, Mass.: Perseus Books.

Ginzberg, Eli. 1992. Economist reflects on osteopathic GME. *The D.O.* 33(1):83–85.

Glass-Coffin, Bonnie. 1994. Anthropology, shamanism, and the "New Age." *Chronicle of Higher Education,* June 15, A48.

Goldfarb, Russell M., and Clare R. Goldfarb. 1978. Spiritualism and nineteenth-century letters. Rutherford, N.J.: Fairleigh Dickinson University Press.

Goldstein, Michael S. 1992. *The health movement: Promoting fitness in America.* New York: Twayne Publishers.

Goldstein, Michael S., et al. 1985. Holistic doctors: Becoming a nontraditional medical practitioner. *Urban Life* 14:317–44.

Goldstein, Michael S., et al. 1987. Holistic physicians: Implications for the study of the medical profession. *Journal of Health and Social Behavior* 28:103–19.

Goldstein, Michael S., et al. 1988. Holistic physicians and family practitioners: Similarities, differences and implications for health policy. *Social Science and Medicine* 26:853–61.

González-Wippler, Migene. 1982. *The santeria experience.* Englewood Cliffs, N.J.: Prentice-Hall.

Gordon, James S. 1984. Holistic health centers in the United States. In *Alternative medicines: Popular and policy perspectives,* ed. J. Warren Salmon, 229–51. New York: Tavistock Publications.

Gordon, James S. 1988. *Holistic medicine.* New York: Chelsea House.

Gordon, James S. 1996. *Manifesto for a new medicine: Your guide to healing partnerships and the wise use of alternative therapies.* Reading, Mass.: Addison-Wesley.

Gordon, Rena J., and Gail Silverstein. 1998. Marketing channels for alternative health care. In *Alternative therapies: Expanding options in health care,* ed. Rena J. Gordon, Barbara Cable Nienstedt, and Wilbert M. Gesler, 87–103. New York: Springer Publishing Company.

Gottschalk, Stephen. 1973. *The emergence of Christian Science in American religious life.* Berkeley: University of California Press.

Gottschalk, Stephen. 1988. Christian Science and harmonialism. In *Encyclopedia of the American religious experience: Studies of traditions and movements,* ed. Charles H. Lippy and Peter W. Williams, 901–16. New York: Scribner.

Gottschalk, Stephen. 1990. Christian Science. In *Christian Science: A sourcebook of contemporary materials,* 5–13. Boston: Christian Science Publishing Society.

Gramsci, Antonio. 1971. *Selections from the prison notebooks.* Ed. Quintin Hoare and Geoffrey Nowell Smith. New York: International Publishers.

Greenwood, Judith G. 1983. *Report on work-related back and neck injury cases in West Virginia: Issues related to chiropractic and medical costs.* Charleston: West Virginia Workers' Compensation Fund.

Greisman, H. C., and Sharon S. Mayers. 1977. The social construction of unreality: The real American dilemma. *Dialectical Anthropology* 2:57–67.

Gross, Martin L. 1966. *The doctors.* New York: Random House.

Grossinger, Richard. 1990. *Planet medicine: From stone age shamanism to post-industrial healing.* Berkeley, Calif.: North Atlantic Books.

Gurin, Joel. 1979. Homeopathy revisited. *Harvard Magazine,* November–December, 12–14.

Hahn, Robert A., and Arthur Kleinman. 1983. Biomedical practice and anthropological theory: Frameworks and directions. In *Annual review of anthropology,* vol. 12, ed. Bernard Siegal, 305–33. Palo Alto, Calif.: Annual Editions.

Hall, Arthur L., and Peter G. Bourne. 1973. Indigenous therapists in a southern black urban community. *Archives of General Psychiatry* 28:137–42.

Haller, John S., Jr. 1981. *American medicine in transition, 1840–1910.* Urbana: University of Illinois Press.

Haller, John S., Jr. 1994. *Medical protestants: The eclectics in American medicine, 1825–1939.* Carbondale: Southern Illinois University Press.

Haller, John S., Jr. 1997. *Kindly medicine: Physio-medicalism in America, 1836–1911.* Kent, Ohio: Kent State University Press.

Hare, Martha L. 1993. The emergence of an urban U.S. Chinese medicine. *Medical Anthropology Quarterly* 7:30–49.

Harner, Michael. 1990. *The way of the shaman.* San Francisco: Harper and Row.

Harrell, David Edwin. 1975. *All things are possible: The healing and charismatic revivals in modern America.* Bloomington: Indiana University Press.

Harrell, David Edwin. 1988. Divine healing in modern American Protestantism. In *Other healers: Unorthodox medicine in America,* ed. Norman Gevitz, 215–27. Baltimore: Johns Hopkins University Press.

Harwood, Alan. 1987. *Rx-Spiritist as needed: A study of a Puerto Rican community mental health resource.* Ithaca, N.Y.: Cornell University Press.

Haug, M. 1975. The deprofessionalization of everyone? *Sociological Focus* 8:197–213.

Henderson, J. Neil, and Kedar K. Adour. 1981. Comanche ghost sickness: A biocultural perspective. *Medical Anthropology* 5:195–205.

Herskovits, Melville J. 1971. *Life in a Haitian village.* 1937. Reprint. New York: Farrar, Straus, and Giroux.

Hess, David J. 1993. *Science in the new age: The paranormal, its defenders and debunkers, and American culture.* Madison: University of Wisconsin Press.

Hess, David J. 1997. *Can bacteria cause cancer? Alternative medicine confronts big science.* New York: New York University Press.

Hessler, Richard M., Michael F. Nolan, Benjamin Ogbru, and Peter Kong-Ming New. 1975. Interethnic diversity: Health care of the Chinese-Americans. *Human Organization* 34:253–62.

Hildreth, Arthur. 1942. *The lengthening shadow of Dr. Andrew Taylor Still.* Kirksville, Mo.: Journal Printing.

Hill, Thomas W. 1990. Peyotism and the control of heavy drinking: The Nebraska Winnebago in the early 1900s. *Human Organization* 49:255–65.

Homola, Samuel. 1963. *Bonesetting, chiropractic, and cultism.* Panama City, Fla.: Critique Books.

Hoover, H. 1963. A hopeful road ahead for osteopathy. *Journal of the American Osteopathic Association* 32:32–45.

Hostetler, John. 1976. Folk medicine and sympathy healing among the Amish. In *American folk medicine: A symposium,* ed. Wayland D. Hand, 249–58. Berkeley: University of California Press.

Hufford, David J., and Mariana Chilton. 1996. Politics, spirituality, and environmental healing. In *The ecology of health: Identifying issues and alternatives,* ed. Jennifer Chesworth, 59–71. Thousand Oaks, Calif.: Sage Publications.

Hultkrantz, Åke. 1992. *Shamanic healing and ritual drama: Health and medicine in native North American religious traditions.* New York: Crossroad.

Huntley, E. E. 1972. Primary medical care in the United States: Present status and future prospects. *International Journal of Health Services* 2:195–206.

Hurston, Zora Neale. 1931. Hoodoo in America. *Journal of American Folklore* 44:317–417.

Ivakhiv, Adrian. 1997. Red rocks: "vortexes" and the selling of Sedona: Environmental politics in the new age. *Social Compass* 44:367–84.

Jacobs, Claude F. 1990. Healing and prophecy in black Spiritual churches: A need for reexamination. *Medical Anthropology* 12:349–70.

Jacobs, Claude F., and Andrew J. Kaslow. 1991. *The Spiritual churches of New Orleans: Origins, beliefs, and rituals of an African-American religion.* Knoxville: University of Tennessee Press.

Jonas, H. S., S. I. Etzel, and B. Barzansky. 1990. Undergraduate medical education. *Journal of the American Medical Association* 264 (7):801–9.

Jones, Bob. 1978. *The difference a D.O. makes: Osteopathic medicine in the twentieth century.* Oklahoma City: Times-Journal Publishing Co.

Jones, David. 1972. *Sanapia: Comanche medicine woman.* Prospect Heights, Ill.: Waveland Press.

Judah, J. Stillson. 1967. *The history and philosophy of the metaphysical movements in America.* Philadelphia: Westminster Press.

Judicial Council to the AMA House of Delegates. 1961. Osteopathy: Special report of the Judicial Council to the AMA House of Delegates. *Journal of the American Medical Association* 177:774–76.

Kao, Frederick F., and Ginger McRae. 1990. Chinese medicine in America: The rocky road to ecumenical medicine. *Impact of Science on Society* 143:263–73.

Kaplan, Bert, and Dale Johnson. 1964. The social meaning of Navaho psychopathology and psychotherapy. In *Magic, faith, and healing: Studies in primitive psychiatry today,* ed. Ari Kiev, 203–29. New York: Free Press.

Kassak, Kassem M. 1994. The practice of chiropractic in South Dakota: A survey of chiropractors. *Journal of Manipulative and Physiological Therapeutics* 17:523–29.

Kaufman, Martin. 1971. *Homeopathy in America: The rise and fall of a medical heresy.* Baltimore: Johns Hopkins Press.

Kaufman, Martin. 1976. *American medical education: The formative years, 1765–1910.* Westport, Conn.: Greenwood Press.

Kaufman, Martin. 1988. Homeopathy in America: The rise and fall and persistence of a medical heresy. In *Other healers: Unorthodox medicine in America,* ed. Norman Gevitz, 99–123. Baltimore: Johns Hopkins University Press.

Kay, Margarita Artschwager. 1977. Health and illness in a Mexican American barrio. In *Ethnic medicine in the Southwest,* ed. Edward H. Spicer, 99–166. Tucson: University of Arizona Press.

Kay, Margarita Artschwager. 1978. Parallel, alternative, or collaborative *curanderismo* in Tucson, Arizona. In *Modern medicine and medical anthropology in the United States–Mexico border population,* ed. Boris Velimirovic, 87–95. Washington, D.C.: Pan American Health Organization.

Kay, Margarita Artschwager. 1993. Fallen fontanelle: Culture-bound or cross-cultural? *Medical Anthropology* 15:137–56.

Kearney, Michael. 1978. *Espiritismo* as an alternative medical tradition in the border area. In *Modern medicine and medical anthropology in the United States–Mexico border population,* ed. Boris Velimirovic, 67–72. Washington, D.C.: Pan American Health Organization.

Keegan, Lynn. 1988. The history and future of healing. In *Holistic nursing: A handbook for practice,* ed. Barbara Montgomery Dossey et al., 57–75. Rockville, Md.: Aspen Publication.

Kelman, Sander. 1971. Toward the political economy of medical care. *Inquiry* 8:30–38.

Kelner, Merrijoy, Oswald Hall, and Ian Coulter. 1980. *Chiropractors: Do they help? A study of their education and practice.* Toronto: Fitzhenry and Whiteside.

Kett, Joseph F. 1980. *The formation of the American medical profession: The role of institutions, 1780–1860.* Westport, Conn.: Greenwood Press.

Kiev, Ari. 1968. *Curanderismo: Mexican-American folk psychiatry.* New York: Free Press.

Kindscher, Kelly. 1992. *Medicinal wild plants of the prairie: An ethnobotanical guide.* Lawrence: University Press of Kansas.

Kirchfeld, Friedhelm, and Wade Boyle. 1994. *Nature doctors: Pioneers in naturopathic medicine.* Portland, Ore.: Medicina Biologica.

Kirkland, James. 1992. Talking fire out of burns: A magico-religious healing tradition. In *Herbal and magical medicine: Traditional healing today*, ed. James Kirkland et al., 41–52. Durham, N.C.: Duke University Press.

Koss-Chioino, Joan D. 1975. Therapeutic aspects of Puerto Rican cult practices. *Psychiatry* 38:160–71.

Koss-Chioino, Joan D. 1995. Traditional and folk approaches among ethnic minorities. In *Psychological interventions and cultural diversity*, ed. Joseph F. Aponte, Robin Young Rivers, and Julian Wohl, 145–83. Boston, Mass.: Allyn and Bacon.

Koss-Chioino, Joan D., and Jose M. Canive. 1993. The interaction of popular and clinical diagnostic labeling: The case of embrujado. *Medical Anthropology* 15:171–88.

Kotarba, Joseph A. 1983. Social control function of holistic health care in bureaucratic settings: The case of space medicine. *Journal of Health and Social Behavior* 24: 275–88.

Krause, Elliot A. 1977. *Power and illness: The political sociology of health and medical care.* New York: Elsevier.

Krause, Elliot A. 1996. *Death of the guilds: Professions, states, and the advance of capitalism, 1930 to the present.* New Haven: Yale University Press.

Kritz, Francesca. 1994. What's covered? *Good Housekeeping,* March, 120.

Kruger, Helen. 1974. *Other healers, other cures: A guide to alternative medicine.* Indianapolis: Bobbs-Merrill.

Kunitz, Stephen J. 1974. Professionalism and survival during the Progressive era: The case of the Flexner Report. *Social Problems* 22:16–27.

Kunitz, Stephen J., and Jerrold E. Levy. 1997. Dances with doctors: Navajo encounters with the Indian Health Service. In *Western medicine as contested knowledge*, ed. Andrew Cunningham and Bridie Andrews, 94–123. Manchester: Manchester University Press.

Kupferer, Harriet J. 1972. Health practices and educational aspirations as indicators of acculturation and social class analysis among the eastern Cherokee. In *Native Americans today: Sociological perspectives*, ed. Howard M. Bahr, Bruce A. Chadwick, and Robert C. Day, 291–303. New York: Harper and Row.

Kyle, Richard. 1995. *The New Age movement in American culture.* Lanham, Md.: University Press of America.

Laguerre, Michel S. 1984. *American odyssey: Haitians in New York City.* Ithaca, N.Y.: Cornell University Press.

Larkin, Gerald. 1983. *Occupational monopoly and modern medicine.* London: Tavistock.

Larson, Magali. 1977. *The rise of professionalism: A sociological analysis.* Berkeley: University of California Press.

Larson, Magali. 1979. Professionalism: Rise and fall. *International Journal of Health Services* 9:607–27.

Lauer, Roger M. 1973. Urban shamans: The influence of folk-healers on medical care in our cities. *The New Physician,* August, 486–89.

Lee, John A. 1976. Social change and marginal therapeutic systems. In *Marginal medicine,* ed. Roy Wallis and Peter Morley, 23–41. New York: Free Press.

Legan, M. S. 1987. Hydropathy, or the water-cure. In *Pseudo-science and society in nineteenth-century America,* ed. Arthur Wrobel, 74–99. Lexington: University Press of Kentucky.

Leserman, Jane. 1981. *Men and women in medical school: How they change and how they compare.* New York: Praeger.

Leslie, Charles, ed. 1976. *Asian medical systems: A comparative study.* Berkeley: University of California Press.

Levin, Jeffry S., and Jeannine Coreil. 1986. "New Age" healing in the U.S. *Social Science and Medicine* 23:889–97.

Levine, Lawrence W. 1977. *Black culture and black consciousness: Afro-American folk thought from slavery to freedom.* New York: Oxford University Press.

Levy, Jerrold E. 1983. Traditional Navajo beliefs and practices. In *Disease change and the role of medicine: The Navajo experience,* ed. Stephen J. Kunitz. 118–45. Berkeley: University of California Press.

Lisa, P. Joseph. 1994. *The assault on medical freedom.* Norfolk, Va.: Hampton Roads Publishing Co.

Lomax, Elizabeth. 1975. Manipulative therapy: A historical perspective from ancient times to the modern era. In *The research status of spinal manipulation,* ed. Murray Goldstein, 11–17. Washington, D.C.: National Institutes of Health.

Lorber, Judith. 1993. Why women physicians will never be true equals in the American medical profession. In *Gender, Work, and Medicine* ed. Elianne Riska and Katarina Weger, 62–74. London: Sage Publications.

Lowenberg, June S. 1989. *Caring and responsibility: The crossroads between holistic practice and traditional medicine.* Philadelphia: University of Pennsylvania Press.

Lowenberg, June S., and Fred Davis. 1994. Beyond medicalisation-demedicalisation: The case of holistic health. *Sociology of Health and Illness* 16:579–99.

Lyng, Stephen. 1990. *Holistic health and biomedical medicine: A countersystem analysis.* Albany: State University of New York Press.

Lyon, William S. 1996. *Encyclopedia of Native American healing.* Santa Barbara, Calif.: ABC-CLIO.

Macklin, June. 1974. Belief, ritual, and healing: New England spiritualism and Mexican-American spiritism compared. In *Religious movements in contemporary America,* ed. Irving I. Zaretsky and Mark P. Leone, 383–417. Princeton, N.J.: Princeton University Press.

Macklin, June. 1978. *Curanderismo* and *espiritismo:* Complementary approaches to traditional mental health services. In *Modern medicine and medical anthropology in the United States–Mexico border population,* ed. Boris Velimirovic, 155–63. Washington, D.C.: Pan American Health Organization.

Madsen, William. 1973. *The Mexican Americans of south Texas.* 2d ed. New York: Holt, Rinehart and Winston.

Marx, Karl. 1978. The German ideology, part I. In *The Marx-Engels reader,* ed. Robert C. Tucker, 146–200. New York: W. W. Norton.

Mathews, Holly F. 1992. Killing the medical self-help tradition among African Americans: The case of lay midwifery in North Carolina. In *African Americans in the South: Issues of race, class, and gender,* ed. Hans A. Baer and Yvonne Jones, 60–78. Athens: University of Georgia Press.

Mattson, Phyllis H. 1982. *Holistic health in perspective.* Palo Alto, Calif.: Mayfield.

McClendon, Nicole. 1994. Hypnotherapy: Reflections of the past. Unpublished paper, Department of Anthropology, University of California, Berkeley.

McConnell, D., P. Greenman, and R. Baldwin. 1976. Osteopathic general practitioners and specialists: A comparsion of attitudes and backgrounds. *The D.O.* 17(12):103–18.

McCorkle, Thomas. 1975. Chiropractic: A deviant theory of disease and treatment in contemporary Western culture. In *The Nacirema: Readings on American culture,* ed. James P. Spradley and Michael A. Rynkiewich, 407–11. Boston: Little, Brown.

McGuire, Meredith B. 1982. *Pentecostal Catholics: Power, charisma, and order in a religious movement.* Philadelphia: Temple University Press.

McGuire, Meredith B. 1991. *Ritual healing in suburban America.* New Brunswick, N.J.: Rutgers University Press.

McKee, Janet. 1988. Holistic health and the critique of Western medicine. *Social Science and Medicine* 26:775–84.

McKinlay, John B., and Joan Arches. 1985. Towards the proletarianization of physicians. *International Journal of Health Services* 15:161–95.

McNamese, Kevin P., et al. 1990. Chiropractic education: A student survey. *Journal of Manipulative and Physiological Therapeutics* 13:521–31.

McQueen, David V. 1978. The history of science and medicine as theoretical sources for the comparative study of contemporary medical systems. *Social Science and Medicine* 12:69–74.

Melton, J. Gordon. 1992. New Thought and the New Age. In *Perspectives on the New Age,* ed. James R. Lewis and J. Gordon Melton, 15–29. Albany: State University of New York Press.

Melton, J. Gordon, Jerome Clark, and Aidan A. Kelly. 1991. *New Age almanac.* New York: Visible Ink Press.

Mertz, Lisa. 1996. The world's oldest profession—touch therapy—and health care policy. Paper presented at the American Anthropological Association Meeting, San Francisco.

Metraux, Alfred. 1972. *Voodoo in Haiti.* Trans. Hugo Charteris. New York: Schocken.

Meyer, Donald. 1965. *The Positive thinkers: A study of the American quest for health, wealth and personal power from Mary Baker Eddy to Norman Vincent Peale.* New York: Doubleday.

Miller, B. W. 1985. Natural healing through naturopathy. *East West Journal* (December):55–59.

Mills, C. Wright. 1956. *The power elite.* New York: Oxford University Press.

Miner, Horace. 1979. Body ritual among the Nacirema. In *Culture, curers, and contagion: Readings for medical social science,* ed. Norman Klein, 9–14. Novato, Calif.: Chandler and Sharp Publishers.

Moerman, Daniel E. 1981. *Geraniums for the Iroquois: A field guide to American Indian medicinal plants.* Algonac, Mich.: Reference Publications.

Molgaard, Craig. 1979. New Age hunters and gathers. Ph.D. dissertation, University of California, Berkeley.

Molgaard, Craig. 1981. Applied ethnoscience in rural America: New Age health and healing. In *Anthropologists at home in North America: Methods and issues in the study of one's own society,* ed. Donald A. Messerschmidt, 153–66. Cambridge: Cambridge University Press.

Mongeau, Beatrice, Harvey L. Smith, and Ann C. Maney. 1961. The "granny" midwife: Changing roles and functions of a folk practitioner. *American Journal of Sociology* 66:497–505.

Montgomery, Scott L. 1993. Illness and image in holistic discourse: How alternative is "alternative"? *Cultural Critique* 25:65–89.

Moore, J. Stuart. 1993. *Chiropractic in America: The history of a medical alternative.* Baltimore: Johns Hopkins University Press.

Moore, John H. 1996. *The Cheyenne.* Cambridge, Mass.: Blackwell Publishers.

Moore, R. Laurence. 1977. *In search of white crows: Spiritualism, parapsychology, and American culture.* New York: Oxford University Press.

Muecke, M. A. 1983. In search of healers: Southeast Asian refugees in the American health care system. *Western Journal of Medicine* 139:835–40.

Murphy, Joseph M. 1988. *Santeria: An African religion in America.* Boston: Beacon.

Murphy, Joseph M. 1992. *Santeria: African spirits in America.* Boston: Beacon Press.

Murphy, Joseph M. 1994. *Working the spirit: Ceremonies of the African diaspora.* Boston: Beacon Press.

National College of Naturopathic Medicine. n.d. *Catalog.* Portland, Ore.

Navarro, Vicente. 1976. *Medicine under capitalism.* New York: Prodist.

Navarro, Vicente. 1986. *Crisis, health, and medicine: A social critique.* New York: Tavistock.

Nelson, Geoffrey K. 1969. *Spiritualism and society.* London: Routledge.

New, Peter Kong-Ming. 1958. The osteopathic students: A study in dilemma. In *Patients, physicians, and illness,* ed. E. Gartly Jaco, 413–21. Glencoe, Ill.: Free Press.

New, Peter Kong-Ming. 1960. The application of reference group theory to shifts in values: The case of the osteopathic student. Ph.D. dissertation, University of Missouri.

Nienstedt, Barbara Cable. 1998. The federal approach to alternative medicine: Co-opting, quackbusting, or complementing? In *Alternative therapies: Expanding options in health care,* eds. Rena J. Gordon, Barbara Cable Nienstedt, and Wilbert M. Gesler, 27–43. New York: Springer Publishing Company.

Nissenbaum, Stephen. 1980. *Sex, diet, and debility in Jacksonian America: Sylvester Graham and health reform.* Westport, Conn.: Greenwood Press.

Null, Gary. 1986. War on chiropractic. *ICA International Review of Chiropractic* 42(2):15–32.

Null, Gary 1998. *Secrets of the sacred white buffalo: Native American healing remedies, rites, and rituals.* Paramus, N.J.: Prentice-Hall.

Numbers, Ronald L. 1978. Do-it-yourself the sectarian way. In *Sickness and health in America: Readings in the history of medicine and public health.* 1st ed. Ed. Judith Walzer Leavitt and Ronald L. Numbers, 87–95. Madison: University of Wisconsin Press.

Numbers, Ronald L. 1992. *Prophetess of health: Ellen G. White and the origins of Seventh-day Adventist health reform.* Knoxville: University of Tennessee Press.

Numbers, Ronald L. 1997. The fall and rise of the American medical profession. In *Sickness and health in America: Readings in the history of medicine and public health.* 3d ed. Ed. Judith Walzer Leavitt and Ronald L. Numbers, 225–36. Madison: University of Wisconsin Press.

O'Connor, Bonnie Blair. 1995. *Healing traditions: Alternative medicine and the health professions.* Philadelphia: University of Pennsylvania Press.

Office of Alternative Medicine. 1992. *Alternative medicine: Expanding medical horizons.* Bethesda, Md.: Office of Alternative Medicine, National Institute of Health.

Oppenheimer, M. 1973. The proletarization of the professional. In Professionalization and social change, ed. Paul Halmos, 213–28. *Sociological Review Monograph* No. 20.

Orion, Loretta. 1995. *Never again the burning times: Paganism revived.* Prospect Heights, Ill.: Waveland Press.

Osherson, Samuel, and Lorna AmaraSingham. 1981. The machine metaphor in medicine. In *Social contexts of health, illness, and patient care,* ed. Elliot G. Mishler et al., 218–49. Cambridge: Cambridge University Press.

Ostgarden, Jo. 1997. Manifested destiny: The new medicine and Dr. Andrew Weil. *Fitness Plus,* September, 5.

Oths, Kathryn S. 1992. Unintended therapy: Psychotherapeutic aspects of chiropractic. In *Ethnopsychiatry: The cultural construction of professional and folk psychiatries,* ed. Atwood D. Gaines, 85–118. Albany: State University of New York Press.

Oths, Kathryn S. 1994. Communication in a chiropractic clinic: How a D.C. treats his patients. *Culture, Medicine and Psychiatry* 18: 83–113.

Pacific College of Naturopathic Medicine. n.d. *Catalog.* Monte Rio, Calif.

Parenti, Michael. 1994. *Land of idols: Political mythology in America.* New York: St. Martin's Press.

Payne-Jackson, Arvilla, and John Lee. 1993. *Folk wisdom and Mother Wit: John Lee, an African American herbal healer.* Westport, Conn.: Greenwood Press.

Peel, Robert. 1988. *Health and medicine in the Christian Science tradition: Principle, practice, and challenge.* New York: Crossroad.

Peterson, Dennis, and Glenda Wiese. 1995. *Chiropractic: An illustrated history.* St. Louis: Mosby.

Pizer, Hank. 1982. *Guide to the new medicine: What works, what doesn't?* New York: William Morrow and Co.

Pizzorno, Joseph E., Jr. 1996. Naturopathic medicine. In *Fundamentals of complementary and alternative medicine,* ed. Marc S. Micozzi, 163–81. New York: Churchill Livingstone.

Poloma, Margaret. 1982. *The charismatic movement: Is there a new Pentecost?* Boston: G. K. Hall.

Poloma, Margaret. 1989. *The Assemblies of God at the crossroads: Charisma and institutional dilemmas.* Knoxville: University of Tennessee Press.

Powers, William K. 1989. The Plains. In *Native American religions: North America,* ed. Lawrence E. Sullivan, 19–33. New York: Macmillan Publishing Co.

Quebedeaux, Richard. 1983. *The new charismatics II.* San Francisco: Harper and Row.

Quigley, W. Heath. 1983. Bartlett Joshua Palmer: Toward an understanding of the man, 1881–1961. *Chiropractic History* 3(1):30–35.

Raboteau, Albert J. 1986. The Afro-American traditions. In *Caring and curing: Health and medicine in the Western religious tradition,* ed. Robert L. Numbers and Darrel W. Amundson, 539–81. New York: Macmillan Publishing Co.

Rayack, Elton. 1969. *Professional power and American medicine: The economics of the American Medical Association.* Cleveland: World Publishing.

Redwood, Daniel. 1995. Interview with Marc Micozzi, M.D., Ph.D. In *Interviews with people who make a difference,* Health World Online. ‹www.healthy.net/library/interviews/redwood/micozzi.htm›.

Reed, Louis. 1932. *The healing cults.* Chicago: University of Chicago Press.

Reid, Margaret. 1989. Sisterhood and professionalization: A case study of the American lay midwife. In *Women as healers: Cross-cultural perspectives,* ed. Carol Shepherd McClain, 219–41. New Brunswick, N.J.: Rutgers University Press.

Reinders, Robert C. 1961. The church and the Negro in New Orleans, 1850–1860. *Phylon* 22:241–48.

Riley, James Nelson. 1980. Client choices among osteopaths and ordinary physicians in a Michigan community. *Social Science and Medicine* 14B:111–20.

Riscalla, Louise Mead. 1975. Healing by laying on of hands: Myth or fact? *Social Science and Medicine* 2:167–71.

Riska, Elianne. 1985. *Power, politics, and health: Forces shaping American medicine.* Helsinki: Finnish Society of Sciences and Letters.

Riska, Elianne, and Katarina Weger. 1993. Women physicians: A new force in medicine? In *Gender, work, and medicine,* ed. Elianne Riska and Katarina Weger, 77–92. London: Sage Publications.

Rivera, G., Jr. 1988. Hispanic folk medicine utilization in urban Colorado. *Social Science Review* 72:237–41.

Rodberg, Leonard, and Gelvin Stevenson. 1977. The health care industry in advanced capitalism. *Review of Radical Political Economics* 9:104–15.

Roebuck, Julian, and Robert Quan. 1976. Health-care practices in the American Deep South. In *Marginal medicine,* ed. Roy Wallis and Peter Morley, 141–60. New York: Free Press.

Romano-V., Octavio Ignacio. 1965. Charismatic, medicine, folk healing, and folk sainthood. *American Anthropologist* 67:1151–73.

Rosch, Paul J., and Helen M. Kearney. 1985. Holistic medicine and technology: A modern dialectic. *Social Science and Medicine* 21:1405–9.

Rosenthal, Saul F. 1986. *A sociology of chiropractic.* Lewiston, N.Y.: Edwin Mellen Press.

Roszak, Theodore. 1969. *Making of a counter culture.* New York: Doubleday.

Roth, Julius A. 1976. *Health purifiers and their enemies: A study of the natural health movement in the United States with a comparison to its counterpart in Germany.* With Richard R. Hanson. New York: Prodist.

Rothstein, William G. 1972. *American physicians in the nineteenth century: From sects to science.* Baltimore: Johns Hopkins University Press.

Rothstein, William G. 1987. *American medical schools and the practice of medicine: A history.* New York: Oxford University Press.

Rubel, Arthur J. 1966. *Across the tracks: Mexican-Americans in a Texas city.* Austin: University of Texas Press.

Russell, P. 1974. *The quack doctor.* Fort Worth, Tex.: Branch-Smith.

St. John, Donald P. 1989. Iroquois. In *Native American religions: North America,* ed. Lawrence E. Sullivan, 133–38. New York: Macmillan Publishing Co.

Saks, Mike. 1994. The alternatives to medicine. In *Challenging medicine,* ed. Jonathan Gabe, David Kelleher, and Gareth Williams, 84–102. London: Routledge.

Saks, Mike. 1995. *Professions and the public interest: Medical power, altruism and alternative medicine.* London: Routledge.

Salmon, J. Warren. 1975. The health maintenance organization strategy: A corporate takeover of health services. *International Journal of Health Services* 5:609–24.

Salmon, J. Warren. 1984. Defining health and reorganizing medicine. In *Alternative medicines: Popular and policy perspectives,* ed. J. Warren Salmon, 252–88. New York: Tavistock.

Salmon, J. Warren. 1985. Profit and health care: Trends in corporatization and proprietization. *International Journal of Health Services* 15:395–418.

Sandoval, Mercedes D. 1979. Santeria as a mental health care system: A historical overview. *Social Science and Medicine* 13B:137–51.

Schafer, R. C. 1977. *Chiropractic health care: A conservative approach to health restoration, maintenance, and disease resistance.* Des Moines: Foundation for Chiropractic Education and Research.

Schiller, Francis. 1971. Spinal irritation and osteopathy. *Bulletin of the History of Medicine* 45:250–56.

Schoepflin, Rennie B. 1988. Christian Science healing in America. In *Other healers: Unorthodox medicine in America,* ed. Norman Gevitz, 192–214. Baltimore: Johns Hopkins University Press.

Scott, Clarissa S. 1974. Health and healing practices among five ethnic groups in Miami, Florida. *Public Health Reports* 89:524–32.

Semmes, Clovis E. 1996. *Racism, health, and post-industrialism: A theory of African-American health.* Westport, Conn.: Praeger.

Sharma, S., and P. Dressel. 1975. *Interim report of an exploratory study of Michigan State University College of Osteopathic Medicine training programs.* East Lansing: Office of Institutional Research, Michigan State University.

Simmons, John K. 1995. Christian Science and American culture. In *America's alternative religions,* ed. Timothy Miller, 61–68. Albany: State University of New York Press.

Singer, Merrill. 1981. The social meaning of medicine in a sectarian community. *Medical Anthropology* 5:207–32.

Singer Merrill. 1982. Christian Science healing and alcoholism. *Journal of Operational Psychiatry* 13(1):2–12.

Singer, Merrill, and Maria G. Borrero. 1984. Indigenous treatment for alcoholism: The case of Puerto Rican spiritism. *Medical Anthropology* 8:246–73.

Singer, Merrill, and Roberto Garcia. 1989. Becoming a Puerto Rican espiritista: Life history of a female healer. In *Women as healers: Cross-cultural perspectives,* ed. Carol Shepherd McClain, 156–85. New Brunswick, N.J.: Rutgers University Press.

Singer, Philip. 1977. Introduction: From anthropology and medicine to "therapy" and neo-colonialism. In *Traditional healing: New science or new colonialism?* ed. Philip Singer, 1–25. London: Conch Magazine Limited.

Siskin, Edgar E. 1983. *Washo shamans and peyotists: Religious conflict in an American Indian tribe.* Salt Lake City: University of Utah Press.

Skrabanek, Petr. 1985. Acupuncture: Past, present, and future. In *Examining holistic medicine,* ed. Douglas Stalker and Clark Glymour, 181–96. Buffalo: Prometheus.

211

Smith, R. 1972. Family medicine and health care crisis in the United States. *International Journal of Health Services* 2:207–15.

Snow, Loudell F. 1973. "I was born just exactly with the gift": An interview with a Voodoo practitioner. *Journal of American Folklore* 86:272–81.

Snow, Loudell F. 1974. Folk medical beliefs and their implications for care of patients. *Annals of Internal Medicine* 81:82–96.

Snow, Loudell F. 1977. Popular medicine in a black neighborhood. In *Ethnomedicine in the Southwest,* ed. Edward H. Spicer, 19–95. Tucson: University of Arizona Press.

Snow, Loudell F. 1978. Sorcerers, saints, and charlatans: Black folk healers in urban America. *Culture, Medicine and Psychiatry* 2:69–106.

Snow, Loudell F. 1993. *Walkin' over medicine.* Boulder, Colo.: Westview Press.

Sokolow, Jayme A. 1983. *Eros and modernization: Sylvester Graham, health reform, and the origins of Victorian sexuality in America.* Rutherford, N.J.: Fairleigh Dickinson University Press.

Spector, Rachel E. 1996. *Cultural diversity in health and illness.* 4th ed. Stamford, Conn.: Appleton and Lange.

Spickard, James V. 1991. Spiritual healing among the American followers of a Japanese new religion. In *Research in the social scientific study of religion,* vol. 3, ed. Monty L. Lynn and David O. Moberg, 135–56. Greenwich, Conn.: JAI Press.

Sprovieri, John. 1993. Teaching OMT: Osteopathic medical schools seek to improve methods. *The D.O.* 34(7):69–78.

Sprovieri, John. 1995. Silencing the critics: D.O.s, Ph.D.s, students answer call to prove efficacy of OMT. *The D.O.* 36(9):49–56.

Stanford Research Institute. 1960. *Chiropractic in California: A report.* Los Angeles: Haynes Foundation.

Stark, Evan. 1982. Doctors in spite of themselves: The limits of radical health criticism. *International Journal of Health Services* 12:419–57.

Stark, Rodney, and William Sims Bainbridge. 1985. *The future of religion: Secularization, revival, and cult formation.* Berkeley: University of California Press.

Starr, Paul. 1982. *The social transformation of medicine.* New York: Basic Books.

Stein, Howard F. 1990. *American medicine as culture.* Boulder, Colo.: Westview Press.

Stekert, Ellen J. 1970. Focus for conflict: Southern mountain medical beliefs in Detroit. *Journal of American Folklore* 83:115–56.

Sternberg, David. 1969. Boys in plight: A case study of chiropractic students confronting a medically-oriented society. Ph.D. dissertation, State University of New York at Buffalo.

Still, Andrew T. 1908. *Autobiography of Andrew T. Still, with a history of the discovery and development of the science of osteopathy.* Kirksville, Mo.: Andrew T. Still.

Studdert, David M., et al. 1998. Medical malpractice implications of alternative medicine. *Journal of the American Medical Association* 280(18):1610–15.

Synan, Vinson. 1971. *The Holiness-Pentecostal movement in the United States.* Grand Rapids, Mich.: W. B. Eerdmans Publishing Co.

Synan, Vinson. 1997. *The Holiness-Pentecostal tradition: Charismatic movements in the twentieth century.* Grand Rapids, Mich.: W. B. Eerdmans Publishing Co.

Tinney, James S. 1978. A theoretical and historical comparsion of black political and religious movements. Ph.D. dissertation, Howard University.

Topper, Martin D. 1987. The traditional Navajo medicine man: Therapist, counselor, and community leader. *Journal of Psychoanalytic Anthropology* 10:217–49.

Toufexis, Anastasia. 1993. Dr. Jacobs' alternative mission. *Time,* March 1, 43– 44.

Traugot, Michael. 1998. The Farm. In *Sects, cults, and spiritual communities: A sociological analysis,* ed. William W. Zellner and Marc Petrowsky, 41–62. Boulder, Colo.: Westview Press.

Trever, W. 1972. *In the public interest.* Los Angeles: Scriptures Unlimited.

Trotter, Robert T., and Juan Antonio Chavira. 1981. *Curanderismo: Mexican American folk healing.* Athens: University of Georgia Press.

Trowbridge, Carol. 1991. *Andrew Taylor Still, 1828–1917.* Kirksville, Mo.: Thomas Jefferson University Press.

Tucker, Cynthia Grant. 1994. *Healer in harm's way: Mary Collson, a clergywoman in Christian Science.* Knoxville: University of Tennessee Press.

Turner, Chittenden. 1931. *Rise of chiropractic.* Los Angeles: Powell.

Turner, Roger N. 1984. *Naturopathic medicine: Treating the whole person.* Wellingborough, Northamptonshire, England: Thorsons.

Twaddle, Andrew C., and Richard M. Hessler. 1987. *A sociology of health.* New York: Macmillan Publishing Co.

Ullman, Dana. 1991. *Discovering homeopathy: Your introduction to the science and art of homeopathic medicine.* Berkeley, Calif.: North Atlantic Books.

Vahle, Neal. 1996. *Torch-bearer to light the way: The life of Myrtle Fillmore.* Mill Valley, Calif.: Open View Press.

Velie, E. C. 1978. *Comparsion of chiropractic and medical treatment of nonoperative back and neck injuries, 1976–77.* Des Moines: Iowa Industrial Commission.

Vespucci, Raffella. 1994. Homeopathy: Ancient wisdom in the twentieth century. Unpublished paper, Department of Anthropology, University of California, Berkeley.

Vogel, Virgil J. 1970. *American Indian medicine.* Norman: University of Oklahoma Press.

Wagner, Melinda Bollar. 1983. *Metaphysics in midwestern America.* Columbus: Ohio State University Press.

Waitzkin, Howard. 1983. *The second sickness: Contradictions of capitalist health care.* New York: Free Press.

Waitzkin, Howard, and Barbara Waterman. 1974. *The exploitation of illness in a capitalist society.* Indianapolis: Bobbs-Merrill.

Wallace, Anthony F. C. 1956. Revitalization movements. *American Anthropologist* 58: 264–81.

Wallis, Roy. 1977. *The road to total freedom: A sociological analysis of Scientology.* New York: Columbia University Press.

Walsh, John. 1972. Medicine at Michigan State (I): Educators and legislators. *Science* 177:1085–87.

Ward, W. Douglas, and Andrea Tomaras. 1985. Colleges of osteopathic medicine: A profile of growth. *Journal of the American Osteopathic Association* 85:719–21.

Wardwell, Walter I. 1951. Social strain and social adjustment in the marginal role of the chiropractor. Ph.D. dissertation, Harvard University.

Wardwell, Walter I. 1965. Christian Science healing. *Journal for the Scientific Study of Religion* 4:175–81.

213

Wardwell, Walter I. 1978. Comparative factors in the survival of chiropractic: A comparative view. *Sociological Symposium* 22:6–17.

Wardwell, Walter I. 1980. The present and future role of the chiropractor. In *Modern developments in the principles and practice of chiropractic*, ed. Scott Haldeman, 25–41. New York: Appleton-Century Crofts.

Wardwell, Walter I. 1982. Chiropractors: Challengers of medical domination. In *Research in the sociology of health care*, vol. 2: *Changing structure of health service occupations*, ed. Julius A. Roth, 207–50. Greenwich, Conn.: JAI Press.

Wardwell, Walter I. 1992. *Chiropractic: History and evolution of a new practice.* St. Louis: Mosby Year Book.

Warner, John Harley. 1987. Medical sectarianism, therapeutic control, and the shaping of orthodox professional identity in antebellum American medicine. In *Medical fringe and medical orthodoxy, 1750–1850*, ed. W. F. Bynum and Roy Porter, 234–60. London: Croom Helm.

Watson, Wilbur H. 1984. Folk medicine and older blacks in southern United States. In *Black folk medicine: The therapeutic significance of faith and trust*, ed. Wilbur H. Watson, 53–66. New Brunswick, N.J.: Transaction.

Weeks, J. 1985/1986. Naturopathic medicine: A northwest renaissance. *Insight Northwest* (December/January).

Weil, Andrew. 1983. *Health and healing: Understanding conventional and alternative medicine.* Boston: Houghton Mifflin.

Weil, Andrew. 1990. *Natural health, natural medicine: A comprehensive manual for wellness and self-care.* Boston: Houghton Mifflin.

Weiss, Gregory L., and Lynne E. Lonnquist. 1997. *The sociology of health, healing, and illness.* 2d ed. Upper Saddle River Falls, N.J.: Prentice Hall.

Weiss, Harry B., and Howard R. Kemble. 1967. *The great American water-cure craze: A history of hydropathy in the United States.* Trenton, N.J.: Past Times Press.

Weitz, Rose. 1996. *The sociology of health, illness, and health care: A critical approach.* Belmont, Calif.: Wadsworth Publishing.

Wendel, Paul. 1951. *Standardized naturopathy: The science and art of natural healing.* Brooklyn: Paul Wendel.

White, Marjorie, and James K. Skipper. 1971. The chiropractic physician: A study of career contingencies. *Journal of Health and Social Behavior* 12:300–306.

Whitten, Norman E., Jr. 1962. Contemporary patterns of malign occultism among Negroes in North Carolina. *Journal of American Folklore* 75:311–25.

Whorton, James C. 1982. *Crusaders for fitness: The history of American health reformers.* Princeton, N.J.: Princeton University Press.

Whorton, James C. 1985. The first holistic revolution: Alternative medicine in the nineteenth century. In *Examining holistic medicine*, ed. D. Stalker and C. Clymour, 29–48. Buffalo: Prometheus.

Whorton, James C. 1986. Drugless healing in the 1920s: The therapeutic cult of sanipractic. *Pharmacy in History* 28:14–25.

Wiedman, Dennis. 1990. Big and little moon peyotism as health care delivery systems. *Medical Anthropology* 12:371–87.

Wiese, Glenda. 1994. Beyond the "Jim Crow" experience: Blacks in chiropractic education. *Chiropractic History* 14(1):15–20.

214

Wiese, Glenda, and A. Ferguson. 1985. Historical directory of chiropractic schools and colleges. *Research Forum* 1(3):79–94.

Wild, Patricia B. 1978. Social origins and ideology of chiropractors: An empirical study of the socialization of the chiropractic student. *Sociological Symposium* 22:33–51.

Williams, Peter. 1980. *Popular religion in America: Symbolic change and the modernization process in historical perspective.* Englewood Cliffs, N.J.: Prentice-Hall.

Williams, Simon J., and Michael Calnan. 1996. The "limits" of medicalization?: Modern medicine and the lay populace in "late" modernity. *Social Science and Medicine* 42:1609–20.

Willis, Evan. 1983. *Medical dominance: The division of labour in Australian health care.* Sydney: Allen and Unwin.

Wilson, Bryan. 1966. The religious teachings and organization of Christian Science. In *Medical care: Readings in the sociology of medical institutions*, ed. W. Richard Scott and Edmund H. Volkart, 41–51. New York: J. Wiley.

Wilson, John. 1978. *Religion in American society: The effective presence.* Englewood Cliffs, N.J.: Prentice-Hall.

Winslow, David J. 1969. Bishop E. E. Everett and some aspects of occultism and folk religion in Negro Philadelphia. *Keystone Folklore Quarterly* 14:59–80.

Withers, Carl. 1946. The folklore of a small town. *Transactions of the New York Academy of Sciences* 8:234–51.

Witherspoon, Gary. 1977. *Language and art in the Navajo universe.* Ann Arbor: University of Michigan Press.

Wohl, Stanley. 1984. *Medical industrial complex.* New York: Harmony Books.

Wolf, C. R. 1979. Industrial back injury. *Congressional Record* S5615–S5616, May 9.

Wolinsky, Fredric D. 1988. *The sociology of health: Principles, practitioners, and issues.* 2d ed. Belmont, Calif.: Wadsworth Publishing Co.

Wolpe, Paul Root. 1985. The maintenance of professional authority: Acupuncture and the American physician. *Social Problems* 32:410–24.

Yoder, Don. 1966. Twenty questions on powwow. *Pennsylvania Folklife* 15:38–52.

York, Michael. 1995. *The emerging network: A sociology of the New Age and neo-pagan movements.* Lanham, Md.: Rowman and Littlefield Publishers.

Zaretsky, Irving I. 1974. In the beginning was the word: The relationship of language to social organization in Spiritualist churches. In *Religious movements in contemporary America*, ed. Irving I. Zaretsky and Mark P. Leone, 166–219. Princeton, N.J.: Princeton University Press.

Zavaleta, Antonio N. 1998. El Niño Fidencio and the *Fidencistas*. In *Sects, cults, and spiritual communities: A sociological analysis*, ed. William W. Zellner and Marc Petrowsky, 95–115. Boulder, Colo.: Westview Press.

Zeff, Jared. 1996. The future of naturopathic medicine. *The Best of Naturopathic Medicine* 1:59–61.

Zellner, William W. 1995. *Countercultures: A sociological analysis.* New York: St. Martin's Press.

Zwicky, John F., et al. 1993. *Reader's guide to alternative health methods.* Chicago: American Medical Association.

Index